Communications in Computer and Information Science 1219

Commenced Publication in 2007
Founding and Former Series Editors:
Simone Diniz Junqueira Barbosa, Phoebe Chen, Alfredo Cuzzocrea,
Xiaoyong Du, Orhun Kara, Ting Liu, Krishna M. Sivalingam,
Dominik Ślęzak, Takashi Washio, Xiaokang Yang, and Junsong Yuan

Editorial Board Members

More information about this series at http://www.springer.com/series/7899

Martina Ziefle · Leszek A. Maciaszek (Eds.)

Information and Communication Technologies for Ageing Well and e-Health

5th International Conference, ICT4AWE 2019
Heraklion, Crete, Greece, May 2–4, 2019
Revised Selected Papers

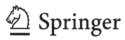 Springer

Editors
Martina Ziefle
Human-Computer Interaction Center
RWTH Aachen University
Aachen, Nordrhein-Westfalen, Germany

Leszek A. Maciaszek
Institute of Business Informatics
Wrocław University of Economics
Wrocław, Poland

Department of Computing
Macquarie University
Sydney, NSW, Australia

ISSN 1865-0929 ISSN 1865-0937 (electronic)
Communications in Computer and Information Science
ISBN 978-3-030-52676-4 ISBN 978-3-030-52677-1 (eBook)
https://doi.org/10.1007/978-3-030-52677-1

This Springer imprint is published by the registered company Springer Nature Switzerland AG
The registered company address is: Gewerbestrasse 11, 6330 Cham, Switzerland

Preface

The present book includes extended and revised versions of a set of selected papers from the 5th International Conference on Information and Communication Technologies for Ageing Well and e-Health (ICT4AWE 2019), held in Heraklion, Crete, Greece, from May 2–4, 2019.

ICT4AWE 2019 received 52 paper submissions from 21 countries, of which 17% were included in this book. The papers were selected by the event chairs and their selection is based on a number of criteria that include the classifications and comments provided by the Program Committee members, the session chairs' assessment, and also the program chairs' global view of all papers included in the technical program. The authors of selected papers were then invited to submit a revised and extended version of their papers having at least 30% innovative material.

ICT4AWE aims to be a meeting point for those that study age and health-related quality of life and apply information and communication technologies for helping people stay healthier, more independent, and active at work or in their community. ICT4AWE facilitates the exchange of information and dissemination of best practices, innovation and technical improvements in the fields of age and health care, education, psychology, social coordination, and ambient assisted living (AAL). From e-Health to intelligent systems, and ICT devices, the conference is a vibrant discussion and collaboration platform for all those that work in research and development and in companies involved in promoting the quality of life and well-being of people, by providing room for research and industrial presentations, demos, and project descriptions.

The papers selected to be included in this book contribute to the understanding of relevant trends of current research on information and communication technologies for ageing well and e-Health. In the next section we would like to demonstrate the diversity of papers, shortly referring to the topics and the research which is addressed in the papers of this book.

The first paper deals with the development of a digital environment for the management of Type 2 Diabetes, in which Vincenzo De Luca and his co-authors report on a novel project, in which the collaboration between public administration and ICT industry for purchasing R&D services is fostered. Telmo Silva, Carlos Silva, and Martinho Mota evaluate iTV companion application and present the results of testing a second-screen mobile application designed for senior users. The project on which the study is based aims at promoting the info-inclusion of Portuguese senior population. Reacting to the importance of good physical conditions and balance control, Christos Goumopoulos and Michalis Chartomatsidis report on the development and evaluation of a new exergame for seniors. The same topic is addressed in another paper, authored by Stephanie Jansen-Kosterink and co-authors, which shows the findings of an iterative evaluation process of mHealth applications for supporting older adults' motivation to stay active. Even though AAL solutions do provide a market of service provision for older adults and their caregivers, yet, public awareness and end-user involvement in

AAL solutions fall short. Rita Tavares Sousa and her co-authors develop a strategy how public attention can be raised for such solutions. Stroke is a common and severe disease not only, but especially for older adults. Peter Mozelius, Karin Ahlin, and Awais Ahmad discuss technology enhanced stroke rehabilitation from a three-fold view of cognitive, motoric, and speech rehabilitation. An author group around Torben Volk-mann and his co-workers demonstrate how older adults can be efficiently integrated as co-designers throughout the development process of a storytelling input component for the Historytelling project, a digital interactive platform for older adults to share life stories across generations. The question on whether technology can support ageing is addressed by Wiktoria Wilkowska and co-authors, by reporting empirically assessed German users' opinions on ageing and use of health-supporting technology. The findings my help to define indicators which contribute to a long-term adoption of medical assistive technology in modern societies. Finally, but not least, in the last paper by Marco Alfano and his co-workers the main characteristics and requirements of online health seeking are demonstrated and a system that allows non-medical experts, but also medical experts, to retrieve Web pages with language complexity levels suitable to their expertise is presented.

We would like to thank all the authors for their contributions and also to the reviewers who have helped ensure the quality of this publication.

May 2019

Martina Ziefle
Leszek A. Maciaszek

Organization

Conference Chair

Leszek A. Maciaszek   Wrocław University of Economics, Poland,
and Macquarie University, Australia

Program Chair

Martina Ziefle   RWTH Aachen University, Germany

Program Committee

Bessam Abdulrazak	Université de Sherbrooke, Canada
Mehdi Adda	Université du Québec à Rimouski, Canada
Carmelo Ardito	Università degli Studi di Bari, Italy
Giacinto Barresi	Istituto Italiano di Tecnologia, Italy
Anupam Basu	National Institute of Technology, Durgapur, India
Karsten Berns	Robotics Research Lab, Germany
Laurent Billonnet	ENSIL ENSCI, Université de Limoges, France
Philipp Brauner	RWTH Aachen University, Germany
Jane Bringolf	Centre for Universal Design Australia Ltd., Australia
Yao Chang	Chung Yuan Christian University, Taiwan, China
Mario Ciampi	National Research Council of Italy, Italy
Georg Duftschmid	Medical University of Vienna, Austria
Stefano Federici	University of Perugia, Italy
David Fuschi	BRIDGING Consulting Ltd., UK
Alastar Gale	Loughborough University, UK
Ennio Gambi	Università Politecnica Delle Marche, Italy
Javier Gomez	Universidad Autonoma de Madrid, Spain
Florian Grond	McGill University, Canada
Nick Guldemond	Erasmus University, The Netherlands
Jaakko Hakulinen	Tampere University, Finland
Andreas Heinig	Fraunhofer Institute for Photonic Microsystems, Germany
David Isern	Universitat Rovira i Virgili, Spain
Eila Järvenpää	Aalto University, Finland
Petr Ježek	University of West Bohemia, Czech Republic
Takahiro Kawamura	Japan Science and Technology Agency, Japan
Jeongeun Kim	Seoul National University, South Korea
Peter Kokol	University of Maribor, Slovenia
Stathis Konstantinidis	University of Nottingham, UK
Andrej Kos	University of Ljubljana, Slovenia

Additional Reviewer

Wendy Rowan   University College Cork, Ireland

Invited Speakers

Nick Guldemond   Erasmus School of Health Policy & Management,
                          The Netherlands
Liz Mestheneos   50+Hellas and Past-President Age Platform, Greece
Miriam Vollenbroek-Hutten University of Twente, The Netherlands

Contents

Developing a Digital Environment for the Management of Chronic Conditions: The ProEmpower Experience of a Horizon 2020 PCP for Type 2 Diabetes

Vincenzo De Luca[1]([📧]) [ID], Strahil Birov[2] [ID], Ozan Beyhan[3] [ID], Simon Robinson[2] [ID], Gorka Sanchez-Nanclares[4] [ID], Maria Del Pilar López Acuña[5] [ID], Adriano Fernandes[6] [ID], Reinhard Hammerschmidt[2] [ID], Giovanni Tramontano[1] [ID], Roberta Patalano[7] [ID], Guglielmo Toscano[1] [ID], Giovanni Annuzzi[1] [ID], Guido Iaccarino[8] [ID], Maria Triassi[9] [ID], and Maddalena Illario[9,10] [ID]

[1] Azienda Ospedaliera Universitaria Federico II, via S. Pansini 5, Naples, Italy
`{ricercaesviluppo.diraup,toscano,annuzzi}@unina.it`,
`giovanni.tramontano@libero.it`
[2] empirica Gesellschaft für Kommunikations- und Technologieforschung mbH, Oxfordstr. 2, Bonn, Germany
`{strahil.birov,simon.robinson}@empirica.com`,
`reinhard.hammerschmidt@posteo.de`
[3] Ministry of Health Turkey, Üniversiteler Mah. 6001. Cad. No. 9, Ankara, Turkey
`ozan.beyhan@saglik.gov.tr`
[4] Servicio Murciano de Salud, Central, 7 Edificio "Habitamia" – 5a, 30100 Murcia, Spain
`gorka.sanchez@carm.es`
[5] FFIS, Luis Fontes Pagán, 9. 1a, 30003 Murcia, Spain
`mpla1204@gmail.com`
[6] Misericordia of Amadora, Innovation Department, Estrada da Portela-Quinta das Torres, Amadora, Portugal
`adrianofernandes@misericordia-amadora.pt`
[7] Dipartimento di Medicina clinica e Chirurgia, Università degli studi di Napoli Federico II, via S. Pansini n.5, Naples, Italy
`robipatalano@gmail.com`
[8] Dipartimento di Scienze Biomediche Avanzate, Università degli studi di Napoli Federico II, via S. Pansini n.5, Naples, Italy
`guiaccar@gmail.com`
[9] Dipartimento di Sanità Pubblica, Università degli studi di Napoli Federico II, via S. Pansini n.5, Naples, Italy
`triassi@unina.it`
[10] UOD Programmazione e potenziamento programmi di Health Innovation, Regione Campania, Centro Direzionale Isola C3, Naples, Italy
`maddalena.illario@regione.campania.it`

Abstract. Demographic change represents the most significant challenge of the 21st century. The aging population around the world will foster a consequent change in labor markets, wealth distribution, request of goods and services, as well as social and healthcare needs. The number of survivors to once deadly

© Springer Nature Switzerland AG 2020
M. Ziefle and L. A. Maciaszek (Eds.): ICT4AWE 2019, CCIS 1219, pp. 1–15, 2020.
https://doi.org/10.1007/978-3-030-52677-1_1

conditions, as well as the age associated increase in degenerative chronic conditions will represent a severe stress to our systems, that will not be sustainable any longer. At the same time, longevity might become an opportunity for the reorganization of services, leading to a new era of opportunities for economic and social prosperity. These challenges require a strong interdisciplinary approach in the identification of unmet needs, and new social, health and technological solutions, that are demand-driven and user-oriented. ICT is going to be the key to many of these revolutionary services. The European Community has proposed a new grant instrument to foster the collaboration between public administration and ICT industry for purchasing Research and Development services in order to develop a novel Information and Communication Technology solution, called Pre Commercial Procurement. ProEmpower is such a project aimed to enable patients to early diagnosis, daily management, and clinical data collection for people with type 2 diabetes. The project goes through a call for tenders issued by a consortium of four public procurers, that jointly defined a set of requirements and use cases, in collaboration with end-users, for the development of innovative solutions This manuscript describes the process that has led to the selection of two solutions that will be tested by end users in the four regions.

Keywords: Pre-commercial procurement · ICT · Technical specifications · Diabetes mellitus · Innovation

1 Introduction

Public procurement is the process by which public authorities - including all levels of government and public agencies - purchase goods and services or commission works. These contracts represent a significant share of the European Union (EU) market, accounting for around 14% of its gross domestic product (GDP) [1, 2]. Horizon 2020, the EU framework program for research and innovation, has introduced two innovative forms of public procurement: Public Procurements for Innovative Solutions (PPI) and Pre Commercial Procurements (PCP) [1].

PPI denotes a procurement procedure in which the contracting authorities act as launching customers for innovative goods and services that are not yet available on a large-scale commercial basis and which may include evidence of compliance. PCP denotes the procurement of research and development services that provide for the sharing of risks and benefits to market conditions and the competitive development by phases, in which a separation of the research phases is envisaged; if the goods or services developed during the research and development phase are to be purchased, this should be based on a separate procurement procedure. Pre-commercial procurement is excluded from the Public Procurement directives and in 2007 the European Commission (EC) developed specific guidelines for Member States explaining how to develop procedures for pre-commercial procurement [2].

Innovative public procurement plays a key role in improving the efficiency and quality of public services and at the same time addressing major societal challenges. They contribute to obtaining the best quality/price ratio as well as broader economic, environmental and social benefits through the generation of new ideas and their translation into innovative products and services, thus promoting sustainable economic growth, to the advantage of European companies and Small and Medium Enterprises [3].

The rising demand for health, social and informal care services, due to the demographic ageing and the growing burden of chronic diseases, coupled with limited public resources for health and social assistance are pushing Member States towards of the digital transformation of health and care in an aging society. At the same time, the massive quantity of generated data sparked the development of new techniques to analyze and elaborate biomedical datasets [4–6]. The development of information technology tools and methods, like simulation models [7, 8] and decision making techniques [9], is helping both clinicians and patients and improving healthcare quality as well as health technology assessment [10–12]. A number of industrial players, regional authorities, professional organizations and multi-stakeholder platforms such as the European Innovation Partnership on Active and Healthy Ageing, created a *Blueprint on the digital transformation of health and care in Europe* [13]. By developing "personas", "use cases", and "scenarios", the Blueprint approach enables a deeper understanding of the target group user's interaction with a particular technology, to guide the design process. [14].

By promoting innovation on the demand side and by orienting the development and the first application of innovative solutions to public and market needs, innovative public procurements can allow customers to avoid the costs deriving from unnecessary functions, prevent lock-in to a single supplier and to take into account the long-term needs of the public sector [15].

Type 2 Diabetes Mellitus (T2DM), once a chronic disease of the West, has now spread to every developing country representing one of the most common chronic diseases whose incidence is increasing worldwide [16]. About 336 million people in the world had T2DM in 2011 with an estimated increase to 552 million of cases in 2030 [17]. T2DM is associated with severe complications that impair the quality of life. Obesity, cardiovascular diseases, weight gain, physical inactivity or a low fiber diet with a high glycemic index have been associated with an increased risk of T2DM [18].

"Procuring innovative ICT for patient empowerment and self-management of type 2 diabetes mellitus" (ProEmpower) is a PCP project, financed by EC's Horizon 2020 Programme, aimed to procure innovative Information and Communication Technologies (ICT) solutions for patient empowerment and self-management of T2DM. The objective of the project is to purchase research and development services in order to develop a novel ICT tool able to facilitate the lives of people with T2DM, supporting them in disease self-monitoring, improving their daily lives and allowing the health organizations to manage their clinical data to prevent diabetes complications. The project involves four public procurers across Europe (Turkey, Portugal, Campania and Murcia) that cooperated to develop detailed specifications for new diabetes management processes supported by fully integrated ICT solutions [19]. All procuring partners are fully committed to large-scale procurement of ICT enabled, patient-empowered and continuous diabetes care, based on the outcomes of ProEmpower.

2   Methods

2.1   A Vision to Guide Requirements

The buyers' wishes have been merged into a common vision within the project. A shared vision document was drafted which identified the building blocks of continuous diabetes self-management. It was rendered as a story using two different view-points – the patient's and the healthcare professional's. The document underwent an extensive review process by consortium members and experts.

2.2   Co-design with Target Groups

To ensure that the system is properly embedded into care processes, working routines and end-users' day-to-day life, ProEmpower includes a co-design work strand running in parallel to all phases of the PCP. This work strand encompasses requirements analysis, iterative development of uses cases and service process models as well as the development and conduction of training activities supporting the necessary change management in each country or region. In terms of requirements elicitation, users are actively involved, through a questionnaire, in identifying needs and providing opinion on possible functions (functional requirements) which are given to them. The questionnaire also includes open questions to capture users' personal expectations of ProEmpower. Users are understood as diabetic patients, healthcare professionals treating them, and informal carers who help patients with their daily diabetes management.

The collected information was used to inform the elaboration of functional, nonfunctional, legal and regulatory requirements. Each requirement was described using ID, name, summary, and priority for implementation.

2.3   Use Cases

A set of use cases and service process models has been developed in ProEmpower. Each use case is described in full detail with one corresponding process model with the same name and ID. Use Case development includes the following activities:

- Identify all the different users of the system;
- Create a user profile for each category of users, including all the roles the users play that are relevant to the system.
- For each role, identify all the significant goals the users have that the system will support.
- Create a use case for each goal, following a use case template (Fig. 2).
- Maintain the same level of abstraction throughout the use case. Steps in higher-level use cases may be treated as goals for lower level (i.e., more detailed), sub-use cases.
- Structure the use cases. Avoid over-structuring, as this can make the use cases harder to follow.

2.4 Business Process Model

The process models follow the Business Process Model and Notation (BPMN) 2.0 open specification maintained by the Object Management Group (OMG) [20]. The primary goal of BPMN is to provide a notation that is readily understandable by all business users, from the business analysts that create the initial drafts of the processes, to the technical developers responsible for implementing the technology that will perform those processes, and finally, the business people who will manage and monitor these processes.

Service process model development includes the following activities:

- For each use case, create a first outline of the process model set based on the developed use cases.
- Refine the process model set based on feedback from the procurers (as by definition BPMN should be understandable and utilized by all business users).
- Create a final set of process models to validate technical accuracy against the BPMN specification.

2.5 Open Market Consultation

In order to develop an open and inclusive dialogue between end users, buyers and suppliers that enable new relevant and user-friendly solutions for the good of patients, clinicians, regions and benefit the participating companies, five Open Market Consultation (OMC) workshops were organized in Ankara, Lisbon, Murcia, Naples and Sofia, and one webinar. The aim of OMC is to create awareness about possibilities for innovative/dialogue based procurement strategies, communicate the challenge to potential bidders, and get input for the tender material and process.

2.6 Call for Tenders

PCP means that public procurers challenge innovative players on the market, via an open, transparent and competitive process, publishing a call for tenders to develop new solutions for a technologically demanding mid- to long-term challenge that is in the public interest and requires new research and development services.

The PCP selection process involves three phases (Fig. 1):

Phase I (Concept Design, Solution Architecture and Technical Specifications) aims to verify the technical, economic and organizational feasibility of the proposals with respect to the pros and cons of potential alternative solutions;
Phase II (Development of Prototype Systems) aims to verify to what extent the main characteristics of the prototype correspond to the requirements indicated by the procurers for the desired solution;
Phase III (Development and Testing of Pilot Systems) aims to verify and compare the efficiency of the solutions in real operating settings, involving the end-users for which they are intended.

The ProEmpower PCP project ends after phase III without procurement at scale. This can be subject to PPI during which procurers aim at the deployment of commercial

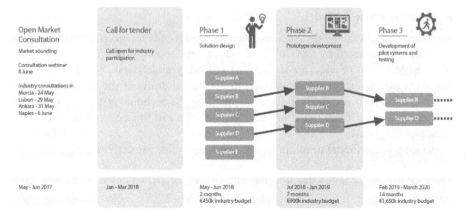

Fig. 1. ProEmpower PCP phases [19].

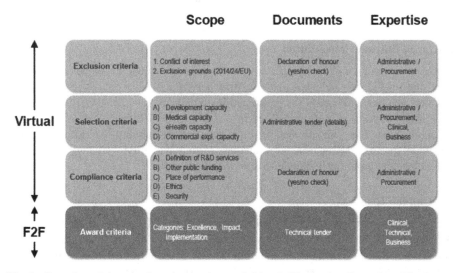

Fig. 2. Overview of the criteria and expertise needed by the Evaluation Committee Members.

volumes of end products and the wide diffusion of newly developed solutions. As this is a separate phase, other suppliers may also enter the competition.

The evaluation of the tenders is performed by an Evaluation Committee which is assisted by an Expert Board. The ProEmpower Evaluation Committee consists of experts from the ProEmpower consortium, on procurement, clinical, technical and business issues. Each procurer nominated three experts to represent them, leading to a total of twelve Evaluation Committee Members.

The Committee applies exclusion and compliance criteria and then evaluates eligible tenders on the basis of the award criteria. Weightings in terms of points and thresholds have been assigned to each of the criteria.

Depending on the phase, the weightings were adjusted, both in terms of points and thresholds, to reflect the characteristics of the PCP phase. Selection of suppliers in each phase was based on a price-quality formula:

$$Score\ for\ tender\ X\ =\ (Cheapest\ Price/Price\ of\ tender\ X\ *\ 100\ *$$
$$Price\ weighting\ of\ 30\%)$$
$$*$$
$$Total\ quality\ score\ (out\ of\ 100)\ for\ all\ award\ criteria\ of\ tender\ X*$$
$$Quality\ criteria\ weighting\ of\ 70\%$$

The result is formally accepted by the Evaluation Committee in face-to-face meetings.

3 Results

3.1 Key Actors' User Stories

Two user stories have been visualized using a diagram (Fig. 3) to represent:

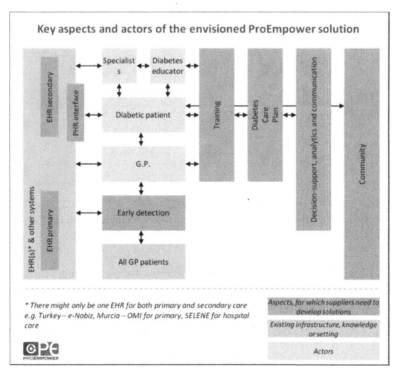

Fig. 3. The ProEmpower vision – diagram.

- the key actors to be engaged in the ProEmpower solution;
- the aspects for which the suppliers need to develop solutions described in a non-technical way as to allow for creativity and innovativeness;
- the existing infrastructure, knowledge and settings the suppliers need to take into account.

ProEmpower is targeting the majority of the population already diagnosed with diabetes mellitus or is in danger of developing this chronic disease. One aim is to close the gap between the onset of diabetes and its detection. Scientific guidelines for the detection of diabetes mellitus and its pre-diabetic states, Impaired Fasting Glucose (IFG) and/or Impaired Glucose Tolerance (IGT), are to be respected (Fig. 4).

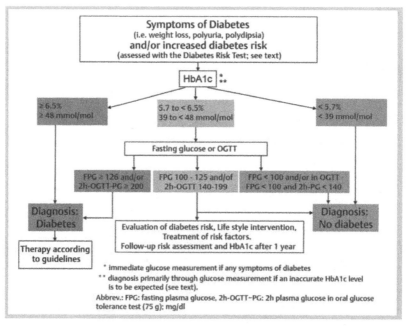

Fig. 4. Diagnostic Algorithm for the diagnosis of diabetes mellitus of the German Diabetes Association [21] in line with IDF [22].

The ICT-based ProEmpower Procurement Solution focuses on supporting patients and medical staff when glucose levels are regularly elevated. This means, persons with IFG and/or IGT are a target audience, besides those with type-2 diabetes. Type-1 diabetes patients and pregnant women are excluded since these patients require different specialized medical care.

3.2 From End-User Questionnaires to Requirements

The questionnaires were finalized in order to collect end-users opinion and translated into Turkish, Spanish, Portuguese and Italian.

The ProEmpower procurers have compiled over 165 requirements for new ICT-enabled diabetes mellitus management solutions for their regions. The requirements were grouped into key topics according to the Chronic Care Model, as shown in Fig. 5.

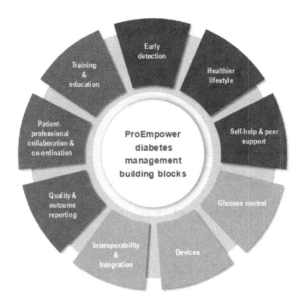

Fig. 5. ProEmpower diabetes management building blocks [19].

3.3 Use Cases and Their Corresponding Process Models

All four procurers took part in the development of common use cases and process models, by nominating dedicated persons to take part in a procurement working group.

The following diagram, in line with the vision of the project, guided the development process (Fig. 6).

In total twelve use cases and their corresponding process models have been defined:

- Enrolling patients into ProEmpower (UC0)
- Integrating data from different sources and ensuring interoperability (UC1)
- Capturing patients' level of knowledge and capabilities (UC2)
- Delivering personalized information using data analysis, monitoring and continuous machine learning (UC3)
- Forecasting daily blood glucose long-term effects (UC4)
- Enabling information exchange through messaging (UC5)
- Coaching on physical activity and nutrition & food for diabetics (UC6)
- Providing diabetes training to patients (UC7)
- Working with a Diabetes Shared Care Plan (UC8)
- Setting and tracking targets (UC8-1)
- Managing events (UC8-2)

FUNCTIONALITIES

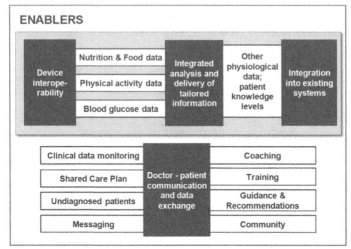

Fig. 6. Overview of ProEmpower aspects which require specification via use cases and process models [19].

- Medication and dose management (UC8-3)
- Generating, viewing and exporting reports (UC8-4)
- Participation in self-help and peer support community (UC9)
- Peer mentoring (UC10)
- Flagging undiagnosed type 2 diabetes patients (UC11)

The ProEmpower solution will differentiate between user types and include new users in the system – physicians, patients, their informal caregivers and other healthcare specialist professionals whose services are required occasionally.

Each procurer will have an overall administrator who can create new physician accounts. Physicians themselves will enroll new patients and their informal caregivers into ProEmpower, as well as include specialist colleagues. The credentials will, as much as possible, re-use existing information and local authentication techniques. They will be used throughout the entire ProEmpower service, including for accessing the Shared Care Plan and the envisioned community platform (UC0).

A key requirement for the ProEmpower solution is that it is interoperable with existing systems and with other devices which are necessary to capture certain physiological parameters. The specific parameter depend on the characteristics of the proposed solution and the data it requires for its algorithms (UC1).

In order to enable personalized information delivery and personalized communication, the ProEmpower solution will process characteristics related to the patient's ability and limitations as well as awareness of and attitude to and diabetes, nutrition and physical activity. By taking standardized tests when enrolled into the ProEmpower solution, patients provide one piece of the necessary data to enable a more personalized ProEmpower service (UC2).

A key expected innovation in ProEmpower is the combination of different data and its monitoring, analysis and processing to deliver personalized decision support to the patient and the healthcare professionals involved (UC3).

The ProEmpower service is expected to make possible a personal in-silico simulation of the patient's blood glucose - insulin interactions based on their glucose-insulin metabolism. This will help achieve a low blood glucose level variation and support the doctor in understanding the patients' long term metabolic profile. It will also sup-port the patient in dealing with travelling and stress, and in adopting a more active lifestyle (UC4).

The different actors in the ProEmpower environment need to be able to exchange information. A question from a patient which requires no more than 30 s to be answered can be more effectively dealt with using a messaging system rather than a live consultation. The ProEmpower solution will make such exchanges possible, but also set meaningful restrictions for the communication. For example, a physician cannot be contacted by a patient at any time or for any reason. The ProEmpower solution will discourage excessive messaging as much as possible, by advising the patient to refer to existing within material the system before a message is sent. There will be clear expectations with regard to the responsiveness of the physician (UC5).

ProEmpower patients will receive comprehensive long-term coaching on nutrition and food choices and ideas which are suitable for type 2 diabetic patients and in line with personal preferences. Harmful effects (such as intolerances and undesired food-drug interactions) will be avoided. Similarly, patients will receive comprehensive long-term coaching on how to prevent and change a sedentary lifestyle (UC6) [23].

After being diagnosed with diabetes, the patient will be given diabetic training at a healthcare facility by professionals. The physician will refer the patient to the diabetes nurse/nurse/diabetes educator depending on their availability. Once a nurse takes over, they will retrieve from the system patient data and more specifically, the level of disease in order to determine which modules/topics should be covered in the training (UC7).

The Diabetes Shared Care Plan will provide the physician and the patient with a common document to help manage the disease. The document will feature a patient interface and a professional interface. The Shared Care Plan represents a structured way in which the patient and their physician can organize the management of the patient's type 2 diabetes. Other actors may be involved as observers (e.g. informal caregivers having an overview of the situation by viewing reports, or specialists who review measured values for different physiological parameters needed for assessment). The document will be accessible online, to be used by the physician during visits, or by the patient at home. The Shared Care Plan will allow to set up and track goals, schedule events, manage alerts and notifications, medication and dosage, as well as view, generate and export reports (UC8). The ProEmpower users (professionals, patients, informal caregivers) will have access to a dedicated community that will foster the exchange of information, peer engagement and regular communication (UC9).

A supportive Community of Practices of end users, distributed in between peer mentors and mentees, will share and exchange experiences, knowledge and other contents related to Diabetes type 2, using different channels such as face-to-face or virtual networks. Peer mentoring, a will establish relationships based on trust between end-users, which will complement the guidance by non-peers (health care professionals) and contribute to enhancing the sustainability and effectiveness to the intervention as a whole. (UC10).

The ProEmpower solution will provide an algorithmic module that uses available existing patient data to identify those patients who may have diabetes type 2. Predictors of diabetes are age, body mass index (BMI), prescribed medication, patient history (family), etc. The identified patients will be flagged, and a list/report provided to the physician in charge of their care. Alternatively, the physician may initiate a request to run the module for a specific patient (e.g. during a control visit) (UC11).

3.4   Results of the Open Market Consultation

A total of 172 companies registered for the OMC workshops. Out of them, 126 different companies attended, accounting for 189 attendees. Most of the attendees came from the procurers' countries: Italy, Portugal, Spain and Turkey, respectively. Regarding the type of companies, most of them where SME/Startups (43%), followed by large companies (31%) (Fig. 7).

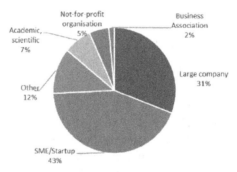

Fig. 7. OMC participants profiles.

3.5   Results of the Evaluation Process

A total of 15 tenders applied to the call for tenders. All electronic submissions were registered and IDs used to ensure smooth operation and efficient discussion among the Evaluation Committee Members. From the 15 tenders, four did not pass the exclusion, selection and/or compliance criteria evaluation. Out of the 11 tenders evaluated on the award criteria, four failed one or more award criteria thresholds and seven were ranked based on the total award score. After applying the quality-price formula, out of the seven remaining tenders, the five highest ranked according to quality-price ratio were within the phase for the budget. Two ranked proposals were not among the winning tenders according to the budget phase limit.

The five awarded solution were:

- **DM4ALL** from a consortium led by GNOMON INFORMATICS S.A. (Greece);

- **DiaWatch** from a consortium led by Tech4Care srl (Italy);
- **CarpeDiab** from a consortium led by Health Insight Solutions GmbH (Ger-many);
- **SHaDE** from a consortium led by Hemosoft Bilisim ve Egitim Hizmetleri A.S. (Turkey);
- **Linkcare** from Linkcare Health Services SL (Spain).

During phase I of the ProEmpower PCP the contractors worked on improving the solution design of the offers made during the call for tenders. The vendors developed in detail the solution design and determined the innovative solutions to be implement-ed during the subsequent phases. They provided details regarding the technical, financial and commercial feasibility of the proposed concepts and explained the approach to be used to meet the procurement requirements. They also incorporated recommendations made by the evaluators in their report. Out of the five offers evaluated on the award criteria, all five met the minimum score thresholds. All five proceeded to being evaluated by applying the price-quality formula after being ranked by award scores. Three supplier consortia have been selected for phase II of the ProEmpower PCP:

- **DM4ALL**;
- **CarpeDiab**;
- **DiaWatch**.

During phase II of the PCP the suppliers produced two versions of prototypes of their systems. The prototype demonstration was conducted in the form of face-to-face meetings between the supplier and each procurer, on the procurers' premises. The pro-curers invited healthcare professionals and patient representatives in order to receive feedback to be used in the evaluation process. The feedback was in the form of answers to a questionnaire (one for patients and one for the healthcare professionals). The results were considered when evaluating the suppliers based on the award criteria (e.g. value of benefits for patients). After applying the quality-price formula the top two highest ranked offers, **DM4ALL** and **DiaWatch**, have been accommodated within the budget foreseen for phase III.

4   Conclusions

Growing public unmet needs and interests require not only innovation in itself, but also innovative ways to trigger, finance and support Research and Development processes until the new products and services that meet these needs arrive to a marketing phase.

Consistent to what happens in the more general scheme of public-private partnership (PPP), the procedural and contractual model of the PCP essentially refers to a form of financing of specific business activities, with consequent sharing of risks and benefits between public sector and Industry. However, the peculiarity and legal complexity of PCP lies in the way in which the contractors are selected and in the regulation of their relations with the public procurer. The greatest advantage that we can derive from the PCP is the strong role of the demand by public procurers in addressing the development of new solutions that can respond to real critical situations, directly ascertained by end users (professionals and patients). The development of a joint call for tenders, that procurers from four countries launched, led the procurers and providers to the challenge of developing a solution that should be adapted to different contexts. In fact, starting from the requirements and use cases set up in the design phase, it emerged that the 4 procurers asked for a solution in 4 languages, interoperable with different levels of sophistication of their IT systems and organizational models.

The functionalities requested by the end users mainly concerned the improvement of the communication between professional and patient, with particular attention to the quality and safety of the data on the clinical parameters of the patients, with the possibility of being able to compare the health outcomes in the medium/long term, between follow-up visits, and patient's empowerment with respect to the disease awareness, medication, nutritional and lifestyles prescriptions.

In addition to the consistency with the identified requirements, an important aspect for procurers for the selection was their ability to provide a solution with increasing levels of maturity, within the time frame established by the call for tenders. The operation and the level of maturity demonstrated during the site visits of the providers made it possible to verify the feasibility of the proposed solutions.

The ProEmpower solutions developed by the two supplier consortia in phase III of the PCP are tackling the challenge of rising incidence rate of diabetes by developing disease self-management solutions that provide a more effective, personalized diabetes management for patients with type 2 diabetes.

The main technical challenges addressed in the solutions are: person-centered care, personalized care, multi-disciplinary care, early detection, personalized decision support, self-management support, self-help and peer support, a learning healthcare system, interoperability and integration.

In conclusion, ProEmpower has already demonstrated the validity of the PCP model for promoting ICT solutions that integrate patient empowerment and healthcare rationalization. The conclusion of the pilot deployment with patient will provide evidences that new models of integrated healthcare supported by ICT are also effective and sustainable.

References

1. European Commission: Horizon 2020 Work Programme 2018–2020: European Commission Decision C(2019)4575 (2019)
2. European Commission: Pre-commercial Procurement: Driving innovation to ensure sustainable high quality public services in Europe. COM(2007) 799 final (2019)
3. OECD: Public Procurement for Innovation: Good Practices and Strategies, OECD Public Governance Reviews, OECD Publishing, Paris (2017)
4. Romano, M., D'Addio, G., Clemente, F., et al.: Symbolic dynamic and frequency analysis in foetal monitoring. In: 2014 IEEE International Symposium on Medical Measurements and Applications (MeMeA), pp. 1–5. IEEE (2014)
5. Improta, G., Romano, M., Ponsiglione, A.M., Bifulco, P., Faiella, G., Cesarelli, M.: Computerized cardiotocography: a software to generate synthetic signals. J. Health Med. Inform. 5(4), 162 (2014)
6. Guarino, F., Russo, M.A., Franzese, M., et al.: A novel shiny platform for the geo-spatial analysis of large amount of patient data (No. e3335v1). PeerJ Preprints (2017)

7. Converso, G., Improta, G., Mignano, M., Santillo, Liberatina C.: A simulation approach for agile production logic implementation in a hospital emergency unit. In: Fujita, H., Guizzi, G. (eds.) SoMeT 2015. CCIS, vol. 532, pp. 623–634. Springer, Cham (2015). https://doi.org/10.1007/978-3-319-22689-7_48

8. Improta, G., Russo, M.A., Triassi, M., et al.: Use of the AHP methodology in system dynamics: modelling and simulation for health technology assessments to determine the correct prosthesis choice for hernia diseases. Math. Biosci. **299**, 19–27 (2018)

9. Santini, S., Pescapè, A., Valente, A., et al.: Using fuzzy logic for improving clinical daily-care of β-thalassemia patients. In: 2017 IEEE International Conference on Fuzzy Systems (FUZZ-IEEE), pp. 1–6. IEEE (2017)

10. Improta, G., et al.: Improving performances of the knee replacement surgery process by applying DMAIC principles. J. Eval. Clin. Pract. **23**(6), 1401–1407 (2017)

11. Revetria, R., et al.: Improving healthcare using cognitive computing based software: an application in emergency situation. In: Jiang, H., Ding, W., Ali, M., Wu, X. (eds.) IEA/AIE 2012. LNCS (LNAI), vol. 7345, pp. 477–490. Springer, Heidelberg (2012). https://doi.org/10.1007/978-3-642-31087-4_50

12. Improta, G., Perrone, A., Russo, M.A., Triassi, M.: Health technology assessment (HTA) of optoelectronic biosensors for oncology by analytic hierarchy process (AHP) and Likert scale. BMC Med. Res. Methodol. **19**(1), 140 (2019). https://doi.org/10.1186/s12874-019-0775-z

13. Blueprint Digital Transformation of Health and Care for the Ageing Society. https://ec.europa.eu/eip/ageing/sites/eipaha/files/news/we4aha_blueprint_update_publishable_version_december_2018.pdf. Accessed 22 July 2019

14. Vincent, C.J., Blandford, A.: The challenges of delivering validated personas for medical equipment design. Appl Ergon. **45**(4), 1097–1105 (2014)

15. Brogaard, L.: Innovation and value in pre-commercial procurement: a systematic evaluation of national experiences. J. Strateg. Contract. Negot. **3**(3), 137–156 (2018)

16. Bommer, C., et al.: The global economic burden of diabetes in adults aged 20–79 years: a cost-of-illness study. Lancet Diabetes Endocrinol. **5**(6), 423–430 (2017)

17. International Diabetes Federation. IDF Diabetes Atlas 8th edition. (2017). www.idf.org/diabetesatlas. Accessed 07 Aug 2019

18. Hu, F.B., et al.: Diet, lifestyle, and the risk of type 2 diabetes mellitus in women. N. Engl. J. Med. **345**(11), 790–797 (2001)

19. De Luca, V., et al.: European specifications for value-based pre-commercial procurement of innovative ICT for empowerment and self-management of diabetes mellitus patients. In: Proceedings of the 5th International Conference on Information and Communication Technologies for Ageing Well and e-Health, ICT4AWE 2019, pp. 19–27 (2019)

20. Business Process Model and Notation 2.0. http://www.omg.org/spec/BPMN/index.htm. Accessed 22 July 2019

21. Kerner, W., Bruckel, J., German, D.A.: Definition, classification and diagnosis of diabetes mellitus. Exp. Clin. Endocrinol. Diabetes **122**(7), 384–386 (2014)

22. International Diabetes Federation Guideline Development Group: Global guideline for type 2 diabetes. Diabetes Res. Clin. Pract. **104**(1), 1–52 (2014)

23. Mann, J.I., et al.: Diabetes and Nutrition Study Group (DNSG) of the European Association. Evidence-based nutritional approaches to the treatment and prevention of diabetes mellitus. Nutr. Metab. Cardiovasc. Dis. **14**(6), 373–394 (2004)

May Technology Support Aging? Diverse Users' Opinions on Aging and Use of Health-Supporting Technology

Wiktoria Wilkowska$^{(\boxtimes)}$ (ID), Julia Offermann-van Heek (ID), and Martina Ziefle (ID)

RWTH Aachen University, Campus Boulevard 57, 52074 Aachen, Germany
{wilkowska,vanheek,ziefle}@comm.rwth-aachen.de

Abstract. Populations of many countries in the world are facing new challenges caused by the current demographic shifts, resulting in a strong increase of the part of society aged 65 years and older. Alongside with economic consequences connected to this phenomenon, societies have to provide improved health care standards, accordingly to the higher needs and requirements of seniors. Assistive technologies (e.g., lifelogging technologies) in the health-related context are capable to support some of the challenges arising from a higher life expectancy and offer more autonomous lifestyle of seniors. However, to be successfully adapted such technologies must be well accepted among diverse potential users. This study examines in an online-survey with $N = 585$ participants current attitudes towards aging and quality of life in old age, as well as indicators of acceptance for health-supporting technologies, which are meant to support seniors and/or persons with chronic disease(s) in their private environments. In addition, this study examines whether user factors like age, gender, and health status significantly affect these opinions. The findings provide valuable insights into these research aims, supporting the understanding of currently changing aging concepts and indicators which contribute to a long-term adoption of medical assistive technology in modern societies.

Keywords: Aging · Medical assistive technology · Technology acceptance · User diversity

1 Introduction

This article is an extended version of a conference contribution [1] and aims under consideration of user diversity at an analysis of current opinions on two important developments which increasingly affect aging societies: the perceptions of aging and the deployment of health-supporting technologies.

Demographic change causing increasing proportions of older people in need of care represents an enormous challenge for feasible and sustainable health care. In more detail, higher proportions of older people – having diverse and specific needs regarding support in line with shortages of care personnel – pose major

© Springer Nature Switzerland AG 2020
M. Ziefle and L. A. Maciaszek (Eds.): ICT4AWE 2019, CCIS 1219, pp. 16–40, 2020.
https://doi.org/10.1007/978-3-030-52677-1_2

economic, political, and social strains for both, the care sectors in specific and the society as a whole [2,3].

Taking Germany as an example, current developments show that a fifth of the population was aged above 65 years and more than a tenth of the population was aged above 75 years of age in 2014. Doing justice also to rising care needs, it has to be considered that almost two thirds of people aged beyond 90 years were in need of care and that the problematic situation of too few people being able to pay and care for seniors is more critical than ever before [4].

The integration of medical assistive technology in everyday life has the potential, on the one hand, to facilitate the professional life of care personnel, and on the other hand, to support older people in being more independent and being able to stay longer at their own home environment. Current developments in the field of ambient assisted living show a broad variety of functions and application potential of single devices, but also complex connected assistive smart home systems, reaching from support of health care by reminding and emergency detecting functions [5], to digital social interaction [6], or facilitating everyday life using automated smart home functions [7].

Besides these technical solutions and their opportunities, the (potential) user's acceptance is a prerequisite for a sustainable usage and integration of assistive technologies in everyday life [8]. Previous research in this field has already shown that the acceptance of assistive technologies differs with regard to specific user groups and their characteristics (e.g., different ages, gender, health status, previous experiences; see Sect. 2.2). Besides demographics, it should also be considered that people's perception of their own person, their aging, and aging itself could be relevant factors for the acceptance of assistive technology. With regard to the perception and mental concepts of aging, research has predominantly focused on the deficit approach, connecting the process of getting older with negative aspects, such as declining skills, loss of mental and physical integrity, or dwindling interests (e.g., [9]). In contrast and with regard to comparably recent research, aging is also considered to be associated with higher optimism, well-being, and higher interpersonal trust [10]. This is in line with the development that older people are increasingly motivated and interested in a healthy living, in shaping their lives actively, and in being more open-minded towards technology with its assistive functions and benefits [11].

Having these changing patterns and ideas of aging in mind, it is of major importance to a) investigate diverse people's perceptions of aging, b) their perceptions and acceptance of using medical assistive technology, c) the impact of different user factors (age, gender, health status) on these perceptions, and d) if the perception of aging relates to the acceptance of medical assistive technology. For this purpose, the current study applied an online questionnaire and empirically investigates a broad sample of (older) participants, having experiences with chronic illnesses.

2 User-Dependent Acceptance of Assistive Technologies

Within the following section, the current state of the art is presented, starting with research on perceptions of aging and acceptance of assistive technology. Subsequently, research on impacting factors regarding the diversity of potential users is summarized. Finally, the research focus and aims of the current study are presented.

2.1 Perception and Acceptance of Assistive Technologies

Future users' positive perception and acceptance are key prerequisites for integrating medical assistive technologies sustainably in the everyday life of (older) people in need of care [8]. Numerous studies in the field of medical technology acceptance approved that the perceptions of benefits and barriers are closely related with the acceptance and intention (not) to use medical assistive technologies.

Most studies conducted in this research field revealed a positive attitude of the participants, acknowledging the technology-related advantages (e.g., [12,13]): In more detail, an increased feeling of safety, a more independent and autonomous life, a longer staying at the own home for older people, and also the relief of relatives (in assistance and care) are mentioned to be the most appreciated benefits of using assistive technology. Nevertheless, some perceived barriers have been proven to be relevant having the potential to hinder the acceptance of medical assistive technologies. On the one hand, the potential violation of the individual privacy represents a severe barrier of using assistive technologies mainly due to aspects such as handling of recorded data, data storage, and the question of who has access to technology- or system-related data (e.g., [13,14]). Other relevant barriers deal with the feeling of being supervised and controlled or the feeling of isolation due to a substitution of human contact and care by technology [15]. In the last years, research in this field showed that the acceptance of medical assistive technology depends on the respective application context and on the specific type of the technology (e.g., [16–18]). Besides these impacting parameters, research has also revealed that the acceptance of medical assistive technology differs with regard to the respective user group and their specific requirements.

2.2 User Diversity as Impacting Parameter(s)

Whenever perception and acceptance of assistive technologies are investigated, the heterogeneity of future users should be considered, because the diversity of users and specific needs and requirements of diverse stakeholders have been proven to influence the evaluation of a specific technology's benefits and barriers as well as the intention to use it in everyday life. In the following, exemplary findings for impacting user factors are introduced.

Gender. Starting with gender, diverse studies found differences between women and men regarding health care, health-related behaviors, and also with regard to the evaluation and perception of using assistive technologies. In the area of health care, it was found that there are gender differences with regard to people's health care-seeking behavior, e.g., women reported to visit their primary care provider more often than men for both physical and mental health concerns [19].

Another study found significant effects of gender on the participants' willingness to use medical technologies to prolong life: Older females opposed to use medical technologies to extend life twice as likely as the male participants [20].

Other studies did not found effects of gender on the participants attitudes towards using medical technology, while interacting effects of age and gender were identified [21,22]. Furthermore, an effect of gender on the participants evaluation of quality of life in older age was found [21] – indicating that aspects like autonomy, social contacts, and caring about health are more important for women than men.

So far, it has not been investigated to which extent gender might have an influence on perceptions of aging related with the acceptance of assistive technology – in particular not with regard to older females suffering from chronic diseases.

Age, Health Status, and Care Experience. In the context of demographic change, it is necessary to consider the participants' age, their health status, potential care needs, and also previous experiences with care as potential influencing parameters on the acceptance of medical assistive technologies.

In the past, several studies investigated the influence of age on technology acceptance (e.g., [14,15,21]). In some of these studies, age had an effect on technology acceptance, indicating a lower acceptance for older participants, whereas in other studies age did not have an effect. Therefore, a study is needed which investigates the impact of age with regard to a large sample of participants of all ages focusing on their perceptions of aging related with their acceptance of health-supporting technologies.

In line with the participants' age, their health status [23], but also potential care needs [24], or previous experiences with care [24,25] were investigated as influencing parameters for technology acceptance. These studies found that the acceptance of assistive technologies differed for user groups having different experiences with diseases and care. For example [24,25], professional caregivers were proven to be the most 'critical' user group – reporting the lowest evaluation of benefits and acceptance and the highest evaluations of barriers (in particular with regard to privacy and data security) compared to other user groups. The results also show [24] that for people with diverse health and care conditions different benefits and barriers of using assistive technologies were relevant for the acceptance and intention to use them. Therefore, these factors should also be considered in an investigation of a broad range of participants with different age profiles.

Perception of Aging. In the past, aging was predominantly associated with negative aspects such as a loss of physiological integrity, "leading to impaired functions and increased vulnerability to death" ([26], p. 1194) affecting almost all aspects of human life. This way, aging was often connected with higher risks of chronic diseases and therefore also with a higher probability of needs for medical assistance or care [27]. These negative effects of aging are opposite to the advantages the usage of medical assistive technology is able to bring – in terms of contributing to aging in place by enabling increased comfort, emergency detection and assistance, or enhancement of autonomy and independence [5].

These partly contradicting patterns of aging show that aging is perceived differently shaped by attitudes, but also societal and social norms. Therefore, it is of utmost importance to investigate people's attitudes and perception of aging as well as their relationships and potential interactions with the acceptance of using assistive technologies. Several studies have focused on these aspects so far. With regard to self-perceptions of aging, people described to feel younger than their actual age; however, the satisfaction with aging was lower for older participants [28]. In addition to that, it was found that the self-image and the perception of aging is affected by diverse aging stereotypes and then again influence attitudes and behaviors [29]. As an example for this, age is usually connected with a lower self-efficacy in interacting with information and communication technology, which means that findings revealed a lower use, a lower ease of use, and also a lower performance in older adults' interaction with technology [30]. However, other studies found that older adults show the willingness and enthusiasm to learn about new and innovative technologies (e.g., [31–33] and that older adults use assistive technologies more often [11]). It should be considered that a responsible design is a prerequisite of technology usage for those older adults and should be aligned with their expectations, ideas, values, and interests. A quantitative study on older participants' attitudes towards aging revealed an overall positive perception of aging [34]: The participants acknowledged positive aspects of aging, such as making plans or being more relaxed, while they rather rejected most of the negative aspects of aging, such as being a burden to others or loneliness. Within this study, influences of user diversity were investigated as well: The results revealed a significant effect of the participants' age on the evaluations, while gender did not have any impact on the participants' attitude towards aging.

To sum up, aging, age stereotypes, and attitudes towards aging have been researched intensively. This is in line with research on the requirements and handling of technology by older people. However, the relationships between perception of aging and the acceptance and perception of medical assistive technology have not been researched, so far.

2.3 Research Focus and Aims

Analyzing the field of (medical) technology perception and acceptance, numerous studies have focused on age as influencing demographic variable (e.g., [14,15, 21]). In contrast, it is questionable whether both, the perception of benefits and barriers as well as the perception of aging, are impacted by people's age, gender, and health status. A second research aim relates to the question, if the perception of aging is connected with perceptions of benefits and barriers as well as with acceptance of using medical assistive technology. Both of these questions have so far not been investigated for a broad sample of older adults, who suffer from chronic illnesses. Therefore, the present study was designed to investigate individuals' current perceptions of aging and their attitudes towards usage of medical assistive technology, aiming for support of seniors or persons with chronic diseases in their everyday lives. For this purpose, an online-survey was conceptualized focusing on persons of different ages, gender and states of health. The applied method and the design of the approach are presented in more detail in the following section.

3   Method

Based on the findings of previous studies [21,34], we designed an online-survey, which was meant to reach a representative sample of the German population. In this quantitative study, we inquired into two main issues: The first focused on the individuals' concepts of criteria perceived as crucial for successful aging, and their opinions regarding different effects of aging itself. The second main issue focused on attitudes towards the use of medical technology in the health-related context, i.e. modern technologies which are increasingly applied in home environments of chronically ill persons, and have the potential to support especially older, and often multi-morbid, individuals in their everyday duties.

3.1   Materials

In the survey, the following three parts can be distinguished: The first part collected socio-demographic information about the participants, such as age, gender, general state of health, professional background, housing circumstances, subjective vitality [35] as well as the (non-)presence of chronic diseases. Participants also reported on their experience with health-supporting devices and provided information about their general technical self-confidence [36].

In the second part of the survey, we collected opinions related to the process of aging. Firstly, we focused on perceptions of criteria that frame a high quality of life (QL) in older age. For this purpose, we used items, e.g., competent medical care, consistent social network, no being a burden to others, and self-supply in the daily living; an in-depth presentation of these items was already presented in [21].

In addition, we gathered the participants' opinions on positive and negative effects of aging in this part of the survey. Table 1, as adopted from [1], includes some examples of the corresponding items. In each case, the participants assessed the respective items using 6-point Likert-scale response format ranging from 1 (= "I do not agree at all") to 6 (= "I fully agree"). A total of nine items were combined into the scale of quality of life in old age and reached a satisfactory internal consistence of Cronbach's $\alpha = .85$. The minimum score to be reached on this scale was 9, the maximum was 45. Furthermore, the scales for *positive* and *negative* effects of aging reached very high internal validities ($\alpha_{pos} = .93$; $\alpha_{neg} = .95$). The scale for positive age effects comprised 11 items (min $= 11$, max $= 66$) and the scale for negative age effects 13 items (min $= 13$, max $= 78$).

Table 1. Examples for items representing the scales of positive (PEoA) and negative effects of aging (NEoA); taken from [21].

Positive Effects of Aging	Negative Effects of Aging
"In my opinion, seniors (today)...	"I'm afraid that in old age...
...are more mobile and independent than 20 years ago."	... I'll be a burden to my family."
...can maintain their health with lots of physical exercises and careful nutrition."	... my dignity could be severely compromised (e.g., in case of severe illness)."
... can cope better with adversity through his/her own experience."	... my cognitive abilities will shrink."
	... I would be less mobile due to health restrictions and, therefore, socially more isolated."
...have much more time for things they always wanted to do."	... I have more to do with medical equipment than with other people."
... have to keep up with the latest developments in order to stay up to date."	... I depend on others."

The third part of the survey focused on perceptions of benefits and challenges applying to the use of health-supporting technologies. A general attitude towards medical technology (AtMT) has been collected, using following items:

- "For me, using medical technology makes sense."
- "I do not want to use medical technology."
- "I can imagine the use of medical technology."

The participants could express their (dis-)agreement regarding these statements on a 6-point Likert-scale, equal to the one already mentioned above in this subsection. After re-coding of the negatively poled second item, the AtMT-scale reached a satisfactory item homogeneity of $\alpha = .74$ with a minimum of 3 and maximum of 18 possible points. This part of the survey also evaluated possible reasons **pro** and **contra** the use of medical technologies. Thereby, the 6-point Likert-scale (1 = full disagreement to 6 = full agreement) was again used. Items used as perceived pros (e.g., control of bodily functions, quick access to health data, rapid warning of critical vital signs, reduction of dependency on others) reached a very high internal consistency ($\alpha = .96$) and the pros-scale reached a minimum of 14 and maximum of 84 possible points. Similarly consistent were the items that identified the perceived barriers (cons) to the use of health-supporting technology ($\alpha = .95$) and the cons-scale ranged from a minimum 15 and maximum of 90 points. The items were presented in detail in [21].

For the acquisition of participants, we used a professional survey panel platform, which enabled to gather a representative sample of German participants. Respondents were paid for participating by the survey panel's institute. The sample's composition and its characteristics are described in more detail in Subsect. 3.3.

3.2   Research Approach

This study aims at two issues which are of great importance for current societal developments: The first one is the reflection of current opinions about the process of aging and the associated life circumstances. The other issue applies to perceptions of the use of health-supporting technologies as a possible solution or support for autonomy and independence in older age. According to the principle of the responsible research and innovation, we studied these objectives considering the users' diversity in order to uncover potential differences between different user groups.

For the statistical analyses, following research variables were chosen:

As **independent variables**, participants' *gender, age* and *health status* are taken into account. Since the relevance of gender was found in the research not only in the context of inequalities in health [37], but also causing differences in health care-seeking behavior [19], it is an interesting characteristic which can be decisive for the potential use of medical assistive devices. In addition, to understand potential differences in the perceptions of diverse concepts of aging, it is useful to ask groups of persons with various amounts of life experience. We therefore divide the sample into three age groups:

- (1) young (<40 years, $n = 201$; 34%),
- (2) middle-aged (40–59 years, $n = 223$; 38%), and
- (3) seniors (≥ 60 years, $n = 161$; 28%).

Moreover, as it is known from previous research [14], the state of health can significantly influence perceptions of the concerned persons. In our statistical analyses we therefore additionally examine, whether suffering from a chronic disease has a significant impact on the respondents' opinions. With regard to the health status, 31% of the survey participants reported to be healthy (H) and 61% of them declared to suffer from chronic illnesses (CI), like for example cardiac arrhythmia, Crohn's disease, thyroid cancer, asthma, anorexia, or multiple sclerosis.

Aspects considered **dependent variables** in this study applied to aging and use of medical technology. We analyze these as constructed scales, which contain various numbers of internally consistent items, as already described in detail in Sect. 3.1. This includes the following scales:

- *Quality of life in old age (QL)*
- *Positive effects of aging (PEoA)*
- *Negative effects of aging (NEoA)*
- *Attitude towards medical technology (AtMT)*

– *Perceived pros* of the use of health-supporting technologies
– *Perceived cons* of the use of medical assistive technologies.

The research design is presented in Fig. 1.

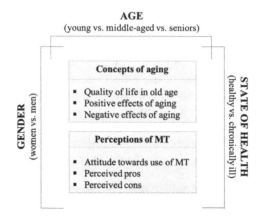

Fig. 1. Research design of the present study (MT = medical technology).

3.3   Participants

Regarding the sample of this study, we intended to cover a broad spectrum of the German population. We aimed at reaching young, middle-aged, and senior males and females, with and without chronic conditions, with different life experiences, educational levels, and professional backgrounds. Moreover, the idea was to encompass individuals with various levels of a general technical self-confidence and experience with the use of medical equipment.

In this study, we collected and analyzed data of $N = 585$ participants, ranging in age between 16 and 84 years ($M = 47.2$; $SD = 16.6$) and 48% of them were females (52% males). As their highest educational levels, participants reported to hold an academic degree (21.5%) and 35.7% completed an apprenticeship. Over 19% of the sample reported to hold a university entrance diploma, and 23.6% a secondary school certificate. Less than half of the sample (44.3%) reported to use and have experience with health-supporting devices in everyday life, like for example with blood pressure meters, blood sugar meters, heart rate monitors, wheeled walkers, and activity monitors.

Different professions were represented in the sample, including engineers, teachers, physiotherapist, economists, psychologists, IT-managers, self-employed businessmen, technicians, caterers, and many more. About 65% of the respondents reported to live together with at least one other person or family, while 35% used to live alone. Choosing statements with regard to the financial situation, 45% of the sample declared "I have to count every penny, but I make ends meet", 46% stated that they're doing relatively well, and around 9% of them reported that they lack nothing in financial terms.

As the empirical study focused on non-invasive and non-clinical research on human subjects and the attendees were transparently informed about the purpose and aim of the intended scientific research, no ethical approval from the ethical committee was sought.

4   Results

For the statistical analyses of influence of the independent variables on perceptions of aging and use of medical technologies, we executed (multivariate) analyses of variance [(M)ANOVA] to examine differences between the age groups (the significance of omnibus F-Tests was taken from Pillai values) and T-Tests for verification of differences between the groups of various states of health. The parameter partial eta squared (η^2) was calculated for effect sizes according to [38]. For continuous variables, Pearson's product-moment correlation coefficients (ρ), and for dichotomous variables Spearman's rank correlation coefficients (r_s), were calculated. For descriptive analyses, the means (M) and standard deviations (SD) are reported in the following. The level of statistical significance (p) was set at the conventional level of 5%.

4.1   Intercorrelations Between the Research Variables

In the first step of the statistical analyses, correlative relations between the research variables were calculated to get a holistic overview over the study data.

The resulting coefficients, as presented in Fig. 2, confirmed strong interrelations between the research variables: A very strong positive correlation was found for perceptions of quality of life and positive effects of aging ($\rho = .72$, $p \leq .001$). The affirmative attitude towards life quality was also positively connected to the perceived benefits of the use of medical technology ($\rho = .64$, $p \leq .001$) and to the general attitude towards MT-deployment ($\rho = .52$, $p \leq .001$). In contrast, the perceptions of reasons against the use of health-supporting technology (cons) correlated moderately with the negative effects of aging ($\rho = .38$, $p \leq .001$) and, correspondingly, inverse with the attitude towards medical technology ($\rho = -.40$, $p \leq .001$). As opposed to that, the latter was strongly positively correlated to the perceived pros ($\rho = .63$, $p \leq .001$).

In addition, for the independent variables age, gender, and health status resulted weak linear relationships with the dependent research variables. The outcomes showed that especially age was significantly connected to almost all study factors. Even when the associations were not very strong, the coefficients indicated that the older the respondents, the more inclined they were to aging and related circumstances of life (QL: $\rho = .14$, $p \leq .001$), and the more positive was their attitude towards aging ($\rho = .23$, $p \leq .001$) and medical technology ($\rho = .16$, $p \leq .001$). Also, with increasing age the perceptions of arguments pro using medical technology were more affirmative ($\rho = .10$, $p = .021$), while arguments

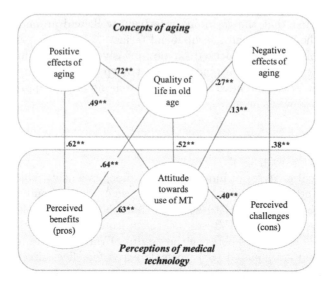

Fig. 2. Correlative relations between the dependent research variables (MT = medical technology).

against its use were more refusing ($\rho = -.15$, $p \le .001$). The correlations are depicted in Fig. 3.

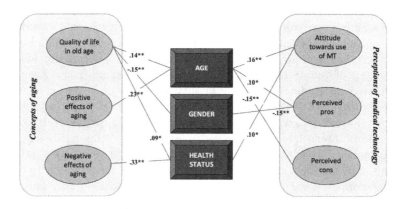

Fig. 3. Correlations between the user factors and dependent research variables.

The correlative relationships for the user factors gender and state of health were less statistically relevant. Gender showed weak connections with quality of life in old age ($r_s = -.15, p \le .001$) and perceived pros of the use of medical technology ($r_s = -.15, p \le .001$) with women having a more positive attitude towards these factors. Correlations regarding the respondents' health condition, and, in particular, the presence of a chronic disease, indicated that individuals suffering from chronic illness tend to be more affirmative to the negative effects of aging ($r_s = .32, p \leq .001$), but on the other side also more positive towards medical technology ($r_s = .10, p = .014$) and high quality of life in old age ($r_s = .09, p = .033$) than healthy persons.

In the next step, the impact of user factors on the dependent research variables will be analyzed in more detail.

4.2   Concepts of Aging

Current perceptions and expectations of aging are the first focused aim of the study. In this section, we examine whether user factors significantly influence opinions regarding high quality of life in old age as well as positive and negative effects of aging. A multiple analysis of variance revealed significant main effects of age [$F(6,1108) = 6.4, p \leq .001, \eta^2 = .03$], gender [$F(3,553) = 6, p \leq .001, \eta^2 = .03$] and status of health [$F(3,553) = 20, p \leq .001, \eta^2 = .10$] as well as interacting effects of age x gender [$F(6,1108) = 2.9, p = .007, \eta^2 = .02$], and gender x health status [$F(3,553) = 3.3, p = .019, \eta^2 = .02$] regarding the concepts of aging. These effects are described more specifically in the following.

Quality of Life in Old Age (QL). Statistic calculations using univariate ANOVA revealed a significant main effect of *age* on aspects accounting for a high quality of life [$F(2,555) = 7.6, p = .001, \eta^2 = .03$]. The respondents of the three age groups differed in their opinions and the young age group reached the lowest means ($M = 41.9, SD = 7.2$) in comparison to the middle-aged ($M = 44.2, SD = 6.9$) and the seniors ($M = 44.4, SD = 5.1$). According to the value of partial eta squared, the effect of age was small-sized. However, despite reaching statistical significance in the differences between the age groups, it is evident that all participants – independently from their age – are very affirmative regarding the aspects of a good quality of life. Figure 4 (left) pictures these differences.

In addition, statistical analysis revealed a main effect of *gender* in the context of QL [$F(1,555) = 15.3, p \leq .001, \eta^2 = .03$]. When looking on the mean scores (see Fig. 4, right), women rated aspects of high quality of life (M = 44.7, SD = 6.3) as more important in older age than men (M = 42.3, SD = 6.9).

Overall, from the descriptive results it can be seen that assessments of aspects accounting for high life quality in older age reach very high mean values, testifying that life quality in terms of autonomy, consistent social life, and competent medical care is an important construct for the 'successful aging'. The state of health, as opposed to age and gender, did not significantly affect the participants' opinions on high quality in older age and no interacting effects were found in this regard.

Positive Effects of Aging (PEoA). Concepts of aging, as operationalized in this study, included also the positive effects of aging. Univariate ANOVA, considering the independent variables *age*, *gender* and *health status* revealed main

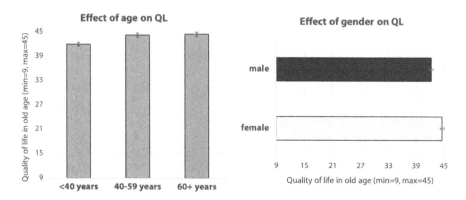

Fig. 4. Main effect of age (left) and gender (right) on the perceptions of quality of life in old age.

effects of age $[F(2{,}572) = 16.4,\ p \leq .001,\ \eta^2 = .05]$ and gender $[F(1{,}572) = 9.4,\ p = .002,\ \eta^2 = .02]$ as well as interacting effect of age and gender $[F(2{,}572) = 3.5,\ p = .031,\ \eta^2 = .01]$ regarding PEoA.

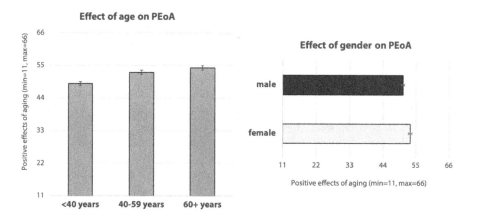

Fig. 5. Main effects of age (left) and gender (right) on the positive effects of aging.

The differences in perceptions of positive aspects of aging between the age and gender groups are depicted in Fig. 5. The senior respondents in the sample $(M = 54.1, SD = 6.7)$ scored with the highest mean values in this regard (middle-aged: $M = 51.9, SD = 10.1$; young: $M = 49, SD = 8.8$), demonstrating that they are the most positive with respect to the process of growing older among their younger counterparts. Considering gender, on average females $(M = 52.2, SD = 8.5)$ are significantly more affirmative in that context than males $(M = 50.7, SD = 9.4)$.

Moreover, we found an interacting effect of age and gender on the PEoA which revealed that female and male participants significantly differ especially in the ages between 40 and 59 years, with male respondents ($M = 49.9, SD = 11.1$) reaching lower means than the female ones ($M = 54.5, SD = 7.7$). The significant interaction of factors age and gender is presented in Fig. 6. Besides, healthy and chronically ill persons did not significantly differ in their opinions regarding PEoA.

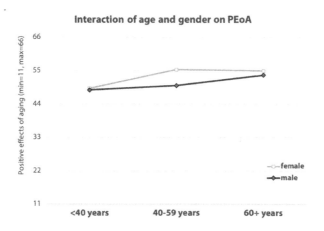

Fig. 6. Interacting effect of age (left) and gender (right) on the positive effects of aging.

Negative Effects of Aging (NEoA). When considering the negative effects of aging as a common scale, statistical analysis of variance revealed significant influences of *gender* [$F(1,572) = 6.5$, $p = .011$, $\eta^2 = .01$] and *health condition* [$F(1,572) = 53.5$, $p \leq .001$, $\eta^2 = .08$] as well as an interacting effect of the both factors [$F(1,572) = 8.3$, $p = .004$, $\eta^2 = .01$]. On the contrary, the effect of age did not reach statistical significance [$F(2,572) = 1.7$, n.s.] and is rather secondary in this context.

According to the effect sizes, especially health status plays a crucial role and the gender differences are less pronounced for perceptions of the negative consequences of aging. The resulting mean values for both factors are presented in Fig. 7 and show that females ($M = 52.8, SD = 13.6$) and most notably chronically ill persons ($M = 54.8, SD = 12.7$) are much more pessimistic with respect to the process of aging than males ($M = 50.4, SD = 13.6$) and healthy individuals ($M = 46.3, SD = 13.4$).

The findings are mirrored in the interaction of the both factors, which is explicitly depicted in Fig. 8. The resulting differences in perceptions of NEoA are evident for healthy individuals, while persons suffering from chronic diseases – independently from their gender – more consistently agree on the negative consequences of aging.

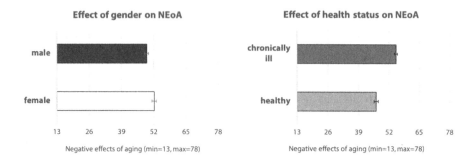

Fig. 7. Main effects of gender (left) and health status (right) on the perceptions of negative effects of aging.

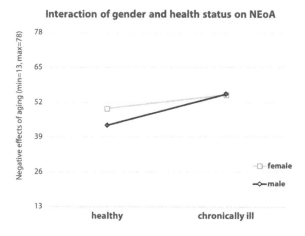

Fig. 8. Interacting effect of gender and health status on the negative effects of aging.

4.3   Perceptions of Health-Supporting Technologies

The second main objective of this study was to gain knowledge about the currently prevalent opinions regarding deployment of health-supporting technologies. In this section, we analyze the influence of the user factors age, gender, and health condition on a general attitude towards the use of medical technology (AtMT), as well as for the perceived pros and cons of its use.

General Attitude Towards MT. An univariate analysis of variance revealed that *age* significantly affects the attitude towards the use and the meaningfulness of medical technology $[F(2,562) = 7, p = .001, \eta^2 = .02]$. According to the effect size the effect was small, but it is easy to see in Fig. 9 that both older age groups of participants (middle-aged: $M = 14.3, SD = 3$; seniors: $M = 14.2, SD = 2.7$) manifested higher values on the scale than the young age group ($M = 13.4, SD = 2.9$). Indeed, a multiple comparison analysis confirms that the differences are significant between the young and the both older age groups, while those between the middle-aged and senior age group are not.

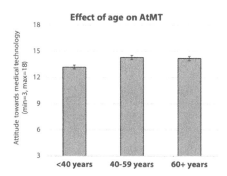

Fig. 9. Main effect of age on the general attitude toward medical technology (AtMT).

Moreover, a statistically significant interaction effect of age and gender $[F(2,562) = 4.8,\ p = .008,\ \eta^2 = .02]$ revealed that attitude toward health-supporting technologies differs between males and females, especially in the young and the senior age group. While the young women scored on average significantly higher than men, in the senior group the mean values invert and the male seniors are more affirmative on MT than the female respondents. The differences are depicted in Fig. 10.

Pros and Cons of the Use of Medical Technology. Eventually, we examined if participants' opinions regarding perceived benefits (pros) but also challenges (cons) resulting from the use of eHealth technologies significantly differ depending on their age, gander, state of health, and/or the interaction between these variables.

For this purpose, we firstly performed a univariate ANOVA for the scale of pros, including all independent variables. The outcomes showed no significant main effects of the user factors on the scale for perceived benefits (pros). The resulting, mostly quite high, average values lie in the upper third of the total scale – a result that approves a high consensus about the numerous advantages of health-supporting technology among the different user groups.

Secondly, the impacts of age, gender, and health condition were examined regarding challenges associated with the use of medical technology, which were summed up to a scale as described in detail in Sect. 3.1. Analysis of variance for the cons-scale revealed a significant impact of *age* $[F(2,564) = 5.1,\ p = .006,\ \eta^2 = .02]$ and *gender* $[F(1,564) = 4.8,\ p = .029,\ \eta^2 = .01]$; these effects are depicted in Fig. 11.

In general, the resulting means show rather little agreement in relation to the perceived contra-arguments and there is a noticeable tendency among the findings: On average, the youngest age group reached in almost all cases the highest

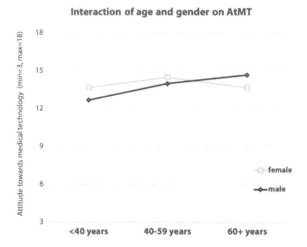

Fig. 10. Interacting effect of age and gender on the attitude towards medical technology.

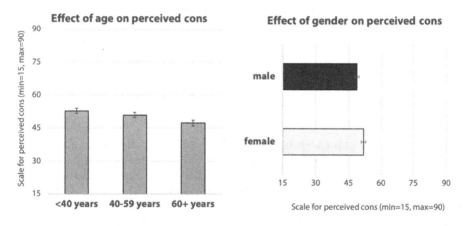

Fig. 11. Main effects of age (left) and gender (right) on perceived cons for the use of medical technology.

values regarding the perceived challenges ($M = 53.3, SD = 14.7$), followed by the means of the middle age group ($M = 50.6, SD = 17.3$). In contrast, the senior age group rather disagreed with these cons reaching a mean of $M = 46.9$ ($SD = 14.3$) out of 90 possible points of the whole scale. This result suggests a higher acceptance of health-supporting technology among the older in comparison to the younger part of the population.

Furthermore, healthy persons and individuals with chronic illness did not differ with regard to the perceived disadvantages of using medical assistive technology. Statistical analysis brought no significant effects for these groups. However, we found an interacting effect of gender and health condition on the perceived cons $[F(1,564) = 14.4,\ p \le .001,\ \eta^2 = .02]$. The joint effect of the independent variables is depicted in Fig. 12: While in the group of healthy individuals female respondents ($M = 54.9, SD = 14.4$) perceive more barriers in using medical technologies than male respondents ($M = 45.8, SD = 14.4$), in the group of persons with chronic illnesses this effect is reversed (females: $M = 49.9, SD = 16.3$; males: $M = 51.3, SD = 15.9$).

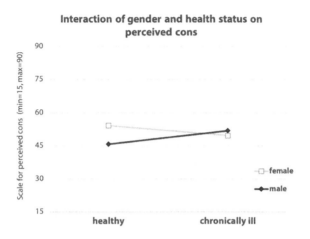

Fig. 12. Interacting effect of gender and health status on perceived cons for the use of medical technology.

In summary, it can be seen that the German respondents have an overall positive opinion about medical assistance technology and this result does not vary in the investigated user groups. The variation of perceptions only becomes apparent in relation to the cons. Younger persons more than older, and women more than man, show a more reluctant attitude in this context, whereby the influence of gender definitely depends on participants' health condition.

5   Discussion

This study is an extension of a conference contribution [1] and aims – under consideration of different user factors (i.e., age, gender, and health condition) – at a reflection of current opinions on two trends which increasingly affect aging societies. The first is the ever growing proportion of seniors in the German population that has been rising sharply, becoming more and more a socio-economic challenge to the country. The second relates to the progressively miniaturized, complex, mobile, sophisticated, and unobtrusive pervasive computing in domestic environments and thus in the private spheres of the residents, which progressively cover different health-related fields with the potential of systematic monitoring of bodily functions. These developments gave rise for this study and were empirically examined in the German population. In the following, we discuss these issues, taking the previously presented findings into account. Thereby, the discussion of the findings clearly focuses on a detailed interpretation of the results and their relationships, while the limitations of the study can be found in [1].

5.1   Aging: A Double-Edged Sword

The consequences of the process of growing older and aspects, which have a direct impact on people's daily life, increasingly penetrate into their consciousness. Since at the latest the beginning of the 21st century, opinions on aging and the associated circumstances have undergone a remarkable transformation. In these fast changing times, not only the thinking about aging (i.e., ideas of who and when is (becoming) old, changing beauty concepts or fashion ideas) but also people's behavior increasingly changes, focusing evermore on "aging well".

The challenges arising from aging societies have been intensively discussed in the scientific community from various points of view (e.g., [39]). One is the economic facet of this phenomenon: In this context, it is not only the fiscal burden connected to rising numbers of older society members, being associated with costs arising from the growing public pension system [40]. But there are also huge costs accounting for provision of health care to the seniors, as with increasing age the need for medical care grows [41]. Further, satisfaction with one's own aging and feeling young have been shown to be indicators of positive well-being in late life [42]. It was also found that negative self-perceptions linked to aging, as associated with physical losses, might impair health-related strategies which are important for maintaining a healthy lifestyle [43].

According to the presented findings, the concepts of aging (as operationalized in this study) gain high attention and the participants principally highly agreed that autonomy and self-supply, competent medical care, consistent social network, and mobility are very important aspects accounting to a high quality of life in older age. In fact, older respondents and the female part of the German sample acknowledged these attributes significantly higher than the younger and the male participants, but overall the examined aspects were judged approvingly for a good life quality. Similar pattern resulted for the perceptions of the positive effects of aging, like for example more time for hobbies or better resistance due to higher experience. This allows the conclusion that people generally highly value such aspects in later stages of life and that the relevance increases with age. Apparently, seniors connote aging less with fragility and decay and see significantly more advantageous purposes in life compared to their younger counterparts; in addition, within the gender groups this is more pronounced for women than men.

In contrast to that, perceptions of the negative effects of aging (e.g., being dependent of or even burden to others, possible loss of abilities and skills) evade the influence of age. In this context, on the one hand, women showed more pessimistic attitudes than men, on the other hand, these aspects were strongly affected by individuals' health condition. Regarding the latter, people with chronic health conditions basically perceived more negative consequences of aging in their everyday lives than healthy persons and, according to the findings, this outcome was independent of the respondents' gender.

To sum up these results, it can be concluded that the process of aging is indeed a double-edged sword: On the one side, there are considerably more possibilities available to us today to age well and healthily. We enjoy ever better medical care and there's a growing awareness of the fact that we can lead our lives into old age on our own responsibility with a reasonable amount of exercise, a healthy nutrition, and a stable social network. On the other side, the process of aging is still strongly associated with increase of (chronic) diseases and various limitations in many areas of life, and to master these poses a major challenge not only for oneself but also mostly for the social environment of the person concerned. Of course, this facet of aging awakens fears and feelings of uncertainty for the own future. At this point, medical assistance technologies can build a bridge between the alleged powerlessness of aging and the new opportunities the use of technology offers. A crucial question now is to what extent are we prepared to allow support in this form and how far are we going to engage in it.

5.2   May the Use of Medical Technologies Support Aging?

A successful adoption of technologies, which are able to support people in their daily lives, is becoming increasingly important to their functional independence [14]. Especially in the last decades technology is unavoidably integrated in many areas of our lives, shaping the ways of how we communicate, work, and perform our daily routine activities [44]. The wide-ranging potential of technical solutions is also increasingly finding its way into the field of health and/or support in the event of illness. This happens not only in the professional context, i.e. in hospitals, in field of care, or in case of special illness, but also increasingly at home even if 'only' in the preventive field.

Being used for health care, assistive technologies offer many possibilities for an autonomous organization of their daily health management, fitness, well-being, and social interaction especially to seniors and/or persons suffering from chronic illnesses. However, to make a real use of the benefits brought by technology development, a certain amount of acceptance for such health-supporting technology is required among the potential users.

The attitude towards technology is an important predictor of technology adoption in the long run [45]. From the previously presented research approach (see [1]) it is known that a positive attitude towards the changes caused by aging comes along with a more optimistic behavioral expectation for an active dealing with its consequences. The good news is that the presented outcomes confirm a quite positive general attitude towards the use of health-supporting technology among the German population and prove that the respondents find such medical assistive technology useful. Our findings indicate that seniors in company with the middle-aged participants are the most enthusiastic group about its deployment and wide-ranging potential. This result may be a little surprising on the one side, because in general younger people are basically more attached to, familiar with, and open to the use of technology. But on the other side, possible explanation for this finding might be that most of the seniors are affected by certain ailments themselves and thus they have a direct relation to the possible use and support brought by health-supporting technology. For the middle-aged the same applies: Maybe in a less direct way, but through persons being either in care or for somebody in need of care they know, such persons can thus highly empathize the real needs and profoundly understand the necessary assistance eHealth can bring.

In addition, the perceptions of pros and cons are regarded as reliable indicators of acceptance. The reasons *pro* of using medical assistive technology are obvious and there is a high consensus about it in the queried sample. The resulting high means in this context indicate agreement on the perceived benefits and this argument is substantiated by the absence of differences between the examined user characteristics, like age, gender, and health condition. In contrast, we found only little approval on opinions regarding reasons *against* the deployment of health-supporting technology in home environments (cons). Furthermore, the opinions significantly varied in the examined age and gender groups: Male and respondents of the senior group reached the least mean values in this context, showing at the same time a high willingness to make use of the potential brought by this technology. In fact, young adults reached on average the highest values, but they still have taken a similarly reluctant position towards the contra-arguments compared to the older age groups. These results do not confirm findings from current studies on general technology and computer use [45, 46], where attitudinal barriers affecting technology uptake among older adults are still higher than among the young ones, and also self-efficacy and behavioral intention indicate a generally lower willingness to use digital technologies among older users. This discrepancy allows at least two possible explanations, as it was already pointed out in the previous research [1]: First, either a long-term adoption of health-supporting technologies is subject to its own dynamics or it testifies that the acceptance of such medical assistive technology in the generation of *today's seniors* have changed. Second, it is possible that acceptance research in the context of medical technology among seniors needs more extended acceptance models (e.g., as the ones used in [47]). For this, further studies are necessary.

According to the correlative relationships of the above presented research variables, a high positive attitude towards the use of medical technology and its perceived usefulness is strongly positively associated with a high quality of life in old age. High positive correlations also resulted for the positive effects of aging and the perceived pros of the technology use, whereas negative coefficient in this regard resulted for the perceived cons. Returning therefore to the question of whether the use of medical technology may or may not support aging, we can therefore confirm – on the basis of the results – that there is a principal willingness and intention to do so, at least in the German population. However, user diversity cannot be neglected when applying health-supporting technology in private environments and the different needs and expectations of the potential users should be carefully taken into account when designing and developing such.

6 Conclusions

Health-supporting technologies, such as medical assistance and health monitoring at home, afford a great potential in the greying societies of today to help to meet the challenges of aging in place. Such applications bring many advantages for the seniors and persons with chronic health conditions and allow an autonomous and active living not only in the later stages of life. This article provides insights into opinions of different potential user groups of the German population, focusing on user factors like age, gender and the health status. The findings support understanding of currently changing aging concepts and point out indicators which contribute to a far-reaching acceptance and, therefore, a successful adoption of health-supporting technology in modern societies.

Acknowledgements. The authors thank all participants for their contribution in the survey. This work has been funded by the project PAAL, funded by the German Federal Ministry of Research and Education (reference number 6SV7955).

References

1. Wilkowska, W., Offermann-Van Heek, J., Brauner, P., Ziefle, M.: Wind of change? Attitudes towards aging and use of medical technology. In: Proceedings of the 5th International Conference on Information and Communication Technologies for Ageing Well and e-Health, pp. 80–91. SciTePress, Crete (2019). https://doi.org/10.5220/0007693000800091
2. Pickard, L.: A growing care gap? The supply of unpaid care for older people by their adult children in England to 2032. Ageing Soc. **35**(1), 96–123 (2015)
3. Deusdad, B.A., Pace, C., Anttonen, A.: Facing the challenges in the development of long-term care for older people in Europe in the context of an economic crisis. J. Soc. Serv. Res. **42**(2), 144–150 (2016)
4. Haustein, T., Mischke, J., Schönfeld, F., Willand, I.: Older people in Germany and the EU. Statistisches Bundesamt, Wiesbaden (2016)
5. Rashidi, P., Mihailidis, A.: A survey on ambientassisted living tools for older adults. IEEE J. Biomed. Health Inform. **17**(3), 579–590 (2013)
6. Delello, J.A., McWhorter, R.R.: Reducing the digital divide: connecting older adults to iPad technology. J. Appl. Gerontol. **36**(1), 3–28 (2017)
7. Demiris, G., Hensel, B.K., Skubic, M., Rantz, M.: Senior residents perceived need of and preferences for smart home sensor technologies. Int. J. Technol. Assess. Health Care **24**(1), 120–124 (2008)
8. Rogers, E.M.: Diffusion of Innovations, 4th edn. The Free Press, New York (2010)
9. Baltes, P.B.: Theoretical propositions of lifespan developmental psychology: on the dynamics between growth and decline. Dev. Psychol. **23**(5), 611–626 (1987)
10. Poulin, M.J., Haase, C.M.: Growing to trust: evidence that trust increases and sustains well-being across the life span. Soc. Psychol. Pers. Sci. **6**(6), 614–621 (2015)

11. Smith, A.: Older adults and technology use. Pew Research Center (2014). http://www.pewinternet.org/2014/04/03/older-adultsand-technology-use/. Accessed 18 Dec 2018
12. Gövercin, M., Meyer, S., Schellenbach, M., Steinhagen-Thiessen, E., Weiss, B., Haesner, M.: SmartSenior@ home: acceptance of an integrated ambient assisted living system. Results of a clinical field trial in 35 households. Inform. Health Soc. Care **41**(4), 430–447 (2016)
13. Peek, S.T., Wouters, E.J., van Hoof, J., Luijkx, K.G., Boeije, H.R., Vrijhoef, H.J.: Factors influencing acceptance of technology for aging in place: a systematic review. Int. J. Med. Inform. **83**(4), 235–248 (2014)
14. Wilkowska, W.: Acceptance of ehealth technology in home environments: advanced studies on user diversity in ambient assisted living. Apprimus Verlag (2015)
15. Beringer, R., Sixsmith, A., Campo, M., Brown, J., McCloskey, R.: The "acceptance" of ambient assisted living: developing an alternate methodology to this limited research lens. In: Abdulrazak, B., Giroux, S., Bouchard, B., Pigot, H., Mokhtari, M. (eds.) ICOST 2011. LNCS, vol. 6719, pp. 161–167. Springer, Heidelberg (2011). https://doi.org/10.1007/978-3-642-21535-3_21
16. Offermann-van Heek, J., Schomakers, E.-M., Ziefle, M.: Bare necessities? How the need for care modulates the acceptance of ambient assisted living technologies. Int. J. Med. Inform. **127**, 147–156 (2019)
17. van Heek, J., Arning, K., Ziefle, M.: The surveillance society: which factors form public acceptance of surveillance technologies? In: Helfert, M., Klein, C., Donnellan, B., Gusikhin, O. (eds.) SMARTGREENS/VEHITS -2016. CCIS, vol. 738, pp. 170–191. Springer, Cham (2017). https://doi.org/10.1007/978-3-319-63712-9_10
18. Himmel, S., Ziefle, M.: Smart home medical technologies: users requirements for conditional acceptance. i-com **15**(1), 39–50 (2016)
19. Thompson, A.E., Anisimowicz, Y., Miedema, B., Hogg, W., Wodchis, W.P., Aubrey-Bassler, K.: The influence of gender and other patient characteristics on health care-seeking behaviour: a QUALICOPC study. BMC Fam. Pract. **17**(1) (2016). Article number: 38. https://doi.org/10.1186/s12875-016-0440-0
20. Arber, S., Vandrevala, T., Daly, T., Hampson, S.: Understanding gender differences in older people's attitudes towards life-prolonging medical technologies. J. Aging Stud. **22**(4), 366–375 (2008)
21. Wilkowska, W., Ziefle, M.: User diversity as a challenge for the integration of medical technology into future smart home environments. In: Human-Centered Design of E-Health Technologies: Concepts, Methods, and Applications, pp. 95–126. IGI Global (2011). https://doi.org/10.4018/978-1-60960-177-5.ch005
22. Wilkowska, W., Gaul, S., Ziefle, M.: A small but significant difference – the role of gender on acceptance of medical assistive technologies. In: Leitner, G., Hitz, M., Holzinger, A. (eds.) USAB 2010. LNCS, vol. 6389, pp. 82–100. Springer, Heidelberg (2010). https://doi.org/10.1007/978-3-642-16607-5_6
23. Klack, L., Schmitz-Rode, T., Wilkowska, W., Kasugai, K., Heidrich, F., Ziefle, M.: Integrated home monitoring and compliance optimization for patients with mechanical circulatory support devices. Ann. Biomed. Eng. **39**(12), 2911–2921 (2011). https://doi.org/10.1007/s10439-011-0407-1
24. van Heek, J., Himmel, S., Ziefle, M.: Helpful but spooky? Acceptance of AAL-systems contrasting user groups with focus on disabilities and care needs. In: 3rd International Conference on Information and Communication Technologies for Ageing Well and e-Health, pp. 78–90. SCITEPRESS Science and Technology Publications (2017). https://doi.org/10.5220/0006325400780090

25. van Heek, J., Ziefle, M., Himmel, S.: Caregivers' perspectives on ambient assisted living technologies in professional care contexts. In: Proceedings of the International Conference on ICT for Aging well, pp. 37–48. SCITEPRESS Science and Technology Publications (2018). https://doi.org/10.5220/0006691400370048

26. Lopez-Otin, C., Blasco, M.A., Partridge, L., Serrano, M., Kroemer, G.: The hallmarks of aging. Cell **153**(6), 1194–1217 (2013)

27. Jaul, E., Barron, J.: Age-related diseases and clinical and public health implications for the 85 years old and over population. Front. Public Health **5**(12), 1–7 (2017)

28. Kleinspehn-Ammerlahn, A., Kotter-Grhn, D., Smith, J.: Self-perceptions of aging: do subjective age and satisfaction with aging change during old age? J. Gerontol. Ser. B **63**(6), 377–385 (2008)

29. Kotter-Grühn, D., Hess, T.M.: The impact of age stereotypes on self-perceptions of aging across the adult lifespan. J. Gerontol. Ser. B **61**(3), 72–77 (2012)

30. Schreder, G., Smuc, M., Siebenhandl, K., Mayr, E.: Age and computer self-efficacy in the use of digital technologies: an investigation of prototypes for public self-service terminals. In: Stephanidis, C., Antona, M. (eds.) UAHCI 2013. LNCS, vol. 8010, pp. 221–230. Springer, Heidelberg (2013). https://doi.org/10.1007/978-3-642-39191-0_25

31. Heinz, M., et al.: Perceptions of technology among older adults. J. Gerontol. Nurs. **39**(1), 42–51 (2013)

32. De Schutter, B., Vanden Abeele, V.: Designing meaningful play within the psychosocial context of older adults. In: Proceedings of the 3rd International Conference on Fun and Games, pp. 84–93. Fun and Games, Leuven (2010). https://doi.org/10.1145/1823818.1823827

33. Knowles, B., Hanson, V.L.: The wisdom of older technology (non)users. Commun. ACM **61**(3), 72–77 (2018)

34. Schomakers, E.-M., Offermann-van Heek, J., Ziefle, M.: Attitudes towards aging and the acceptance of ICT for aging in place. In: Zhou, J., Salvendy, G. (eds.) ITAP 2018. LNCS, vol. 10926, pp. 149–169. Springer, Cham (2018). https://doi.org/10.1007/978-3-319-92034-4_12

35. Ryan, R.M., Frederick, C.: On energy, personality, and health: subjective vitality as a dynamic reflection of well-being. J. Pers. **65**(3), 529–565 (1997)

36. Beier, G.: Kontrollüberzeugungen im Umgang mit Technik [Locus of control when interacting with technology]. Rep. Psychol. **24**(9), 684–693 (1999)

37. Brown, T.H., Richardson, L.J., Hargrove, T.W., Thomas, C.S.: Using multiple-hierarchy stratification and life course approaches to understand health inequalities: the intersecting consequences of race, gender, SES, and age. J. Health Soc. Behav. **57**(2), 200–222 (2016). https://doi.org/10.1177/0022146516645165

38. Cohen, J.: Statistical Power Analysis for the Behavioral Sciences, 2nd edn. Academic Press, New York (1988)

39. Uhlenberg, P.: International Handbook of Population Aging, 1st edn. Springer, Dordrecht (2009). https://doi.org/10.1007/978-1-4020-8356-3

40. Bloom, D.E., Boersch-Supan, A., McGee, P., Seike, A., et al.: Population aging: facts, challenges, and responses. Benefits Compens. Int. **41**(1), 22 (2011)

41. Bosworth, B.P., Burtless, G.: Aging Societies: The Global Dimension. Brookings Institution Press, Washington, D.C. (1998)

42. Kotter-Grühn, D., Kleinspehn-Ammerlahn, A., Gerstorf, D., Smith, J.: Self-perceptions of aging predict mortality and change with approaching death: 16-year longitudinal results from the Berlin Aging Study. Psychol. Aging **24**(3), 654–667 (2009)

43. Wurm, S., Warner, L.M., Ziegelmann, J.P., Wolff, J.K., Schüz, B.: How do negative self-perceptions of aging become a self-fulfilling prophecy? Psychol. Aging **28**(4), 1088–1097 (2013)

44. Boot, W., Charness, N., Czaja, S., Rogers, W., Sharit, J.: Aging and leisure activities: opportunities and design challenges. Innov. Aging **2**(1), 213 (2018)

45. Lee, C.C., et al.: Attitudes toward computers across adulthood from 1994 to 2013. Gerontologist **59**(1), 22–33 (2018)

46. Mitzner, T.L., et al.: Technology adoption by older adults: findings from the prism trial. Gerontologist **59**(1), 34–44 (2018)

47. Chen, K., Chan, A.H.S.: Gerontechnology acceptance by elderly Hong Kong Chinese: a senior technology acceptance model (STAM). Ergonomics **57**(5), 635–652 (2014)

Advisory on Ambient Assisted Living Solutions: Towards an Advisor Concept and Training Curriculum

Rita Tavares de Sousa[1,2]([⊠]), Soraia Teles[1,2], Diotima Bertel[3], Paul Schmitter[4], and Diogo Abrantes[2,5]

[1] Institute for the Biomedical Sciences Abel Salazar, University of Porto, Porto, Portugal
rita.tavaresdesousa@gmail.com

[2] Center for Health Technology and Services Research (CINTESIS), R. Dr. Plácido da Costa, 4200-450 Porto, Portugal

[3] SYNYO GmbH, Otto-Bauer- Gase 5/14, 1060 Vienna, Austria

[4] Zurich University of Applied Sciences, Campus Grüental, 8820 Waedenswill, Zurich, Switzerland

[5] Faculdade de Medicina, University of Porto, Porto, Portugal

Abstract. Ambient Assisted Living (AAL) solutions have opened up a market of service provision for older adults and their caregivers. Insufficient public awareness and end-user involvement on AAL solutions have been influencing the market negatively. Advisory services on AAL solutions are a promising strategy to address those challenges but those are typically missing, provided at a very small scale or by the providers in the context of sales activities. This study aims to identify the prospective benefits of an advisor on AAL solutions, as well as the profile, knowledge and skills required for this role and training preferences. A qualitative study was performed resorting to workshops and interviews with AAL stakeholders to collect data. A comprehensive literature review was carried out to identify experiences and practices on education for AAL advisors. Both data were subjected to a content analysis. Findings were used to define and refine the concept of Authorised Active Advisors, resulting in a clarification of its added-value, on the definition of advisor profiles, as well as on a list of skills and knowledge required. Training preferences revealed by the participants together with the literature analysis, feed a training concept presented in this paper. Finally, the training objectives, contents, learning outcomes and learning/teaching methods are defined and a training hub mock-up is shown. The preferred training modality is based on a blended-learning approach.

Keywords: Ambient Assisted Living · Advisory services · Education and training

1 Introduction

In the last decades, well-known societal challenges posed by the phenomena of population ageing have been propelling the development of innovative solutions such as

© Springer Nature Switzerland AG 2020
M. Ziefle and L. A. Maciaszek (Eds.): ICT4AWE 2019, CCIS 1219, pp. 41–61, 2020.
https://doi.org/10.1007/978-3-030-52677-1_3

products and services based on Information and Communication Technologies (ICT). In particular, Ambient Assisted Living (AAL) solutions have opened up an important market of service provision for older adults and their caregivers. AAL as a concept corresponds to a new paradigm, building on ubiquitous computing devices and new interaction forms targeted at improving older adults health, autonomy, social integration and security [44]. Currently defined as an umbrella market, the AAL market consists of a large collection of products and services in a wide variety of application fields (e.g. health, participation in social life, employment) [1].

In spite of the growing importance of AAL solutions for independent ageing, previous reports highlight the fact that services within this market are often provided in isolation and in a technocentric way [4, 8, 43]. A lack of public awareness on AAL solutions, as well as insufficient end-user involvement, influence the market negatively and contribute most likely to the existing gap between technology development and its uptake by the intended end users [1, 13, 31, 37]. In fact, many care services providers are unfamiliar with technologies that could make their work easier while, at the same time, providers of technological devices and systems are not often aware of what care providers need. The offer of high-quality advisory services for end users on AAL solutions was previously identified as a promising strategy to minimize the mentioned constraints and to promote consumers uptake of such technologies [8]. Yet, the provision of such services is either missing, provided at a very small scale, or offered by product and service providers in the scope of their sales activities [8, 41, 43].

Investing in ICT solutions to increase the scale of advisory services through the creation of a digital neutral/exempt advisory platform on AAL solutions was previously recognized by AAL stakeholders as a potential solution to address those issues [43]. However, previous research from a platform mapping and analysis concluded that personalised feedback and/or advice is generally missing on websites, portals or platforms currently promoting assistive technologies and services for older adults [27]. Moreover, since the consumer journey is growing in complexity in most service sectors, we have, nowadays, rather complex service logics to consider [38]. It was previously argued that both user experience and user empowerment are more likely to be improved when both physical and virtual touchpoints are integrated into service provision [15]. Such integrated service logics would allow taking advantage of virtual engagement in service provision while at the same time minimizing the drawbacks from lack of physical engagement. This market landscape emphasizes the need for trained specialists who can provide knowledge and advice about AAL. The innovations in the field of AAL need professionals, who know how to incorporate, install, maintain, and use AAL products. However, there is no tradition on specific vocational or lifelong training courses in European countries related to the use and development of AAL systems and tools [36].

This paper builds on previous research carried out in the scope of the EU funded ActiveAdvice project, aiming to set up a digital, pan-European advisory and decision-support platform that brings together the broad range of available AAL products, services, and stakeholders. The project is based on the premise that, in the AAL field, an engagement platform must empower stakeholders and facilitate co-creation of value. In this sense, the project outlined the concept of Authorised Active Advisors as a human addition to the digital advisory platform [8, 42]. This paper aims to refine the concept, by identifying the benefits, the profile, and the required knowledge and skills of Authorised Active Advisors.

To fulfil this goal, a qualitative study was carried out aiming at answering the following set of research questions: (i) Are there any good practices on training advisors for AAL solutions? Which ones?; (ii) What are the prospective benefits of an advisor on AAL solutions, and their addition to a digital advisory platform?; iii. What should be the profile of this advisor?; (iii) What kind of knowledge and skills are needed to become an advisor on AAL solutions?; and (iv) How should the necessary knowledge be delivered and the skills trained (i.e. for which training concept are potential advisors looking?). In addition, a comprehensive literature review was carried out to identify experiences and practices (if available) on education and professional specialization for AAL advisors. As an outcome of this work, the concept of Authorised Active Advisor is refined and a training course outline was developed to endow these advisors of such skills and is presented in this paper.

2   Conceptual Considerations

This section will briefly explore two main topics which are of relevance to frame the concept of Authorised Active Advisors, as previously proposed by the authors [8]: (i) the importance of an integrated service logic for AAL advisory services, and (ii) the role of face-to-face advice in the context of a digital advisory platform.

2.1   An Integrated Service Logic for AAL Advisory Services

In recent years, digital service providers have been expanding their portfolio from entirely virtual into the realm of additional physical experience. Thus, we can observe a trend of shifting back from a purely digital to a physical/face-to-face (f2f) interaction, following an integrated logic which makes use of both virtual and physical interaction forms [8, 15].

As previously discussed by the authors [8, 42, 43] there are three main arguments favouring such an integrated service logic for AAL advisory services. First, there is trust. Trust is one of the most critical issues when it comes to the interaction between the consumer and the service provider [10]. Moreover, it is one of the main reasons to invest in an integrated model in service provision, as f2f interaction is perceived as more trustworthy [43]. These arguments hold special relevance for the AAL market since AAL solutions are frequently related to health-related needs. In this sense, data security and privacy acquire increased relevance and the fear of getting low quality, biased or misleading information from non-reliable or exempt sources tends to be more evident [30, 43].

Second, advice on AAL solutions is usually complex. It occurs in a context where interoperability problems still prevail and where no broad and comprehensive information about products, services, and providers is yet available for consumers. Previous reports show that consultation on AAL solutions does happen online, but is usually limited to a first consultancy. Ongoing advice is usually searched in the physical sphere, which is perceived as more trustworthy [43].

Third, although older adults are a quite heterogeneous group which could be per se an argument for a service logic that offers two interaction interfaces as they are still often unfamiliar with technology. Lack of confidence using online channels, and the personal readiness to accept technological solutions depends on many individual aspects such as education, age, gender, physical, mental and cognitive skills, expectations or biographical experience. So, even if barriers associated with ICT skills are expected to decrease in future generations [39], an integrated logic for AAL advisory services might be better able to accommodate future trends. Therefore, the digital advisory platform under development within the ActiveAdvice project cannot be a stand-alone solution [43]. Rather, it must be part of an integrated and systematic service logic, incorporating both virtual and physical services and promoting the integration of different actors with diverse interests and contributions. Authorised Active Advisors should provide the conditions to integrate both virtual and physical dimensions in an optimal solution for AAL advisory services.

2.2 Personal Advice in a Digital Advisory Platform

The concept of Authorised Active Advisor [8, 12] sustains on the premises that a human addition to a digital AAL advisory platform can help increasing personalization in AAL services, empower the consumers in making decisions, enhance trust in AAL advisory and encourage older adults to participate in digital communities, also contributing to the minimization of the digital divide still affecting this age group.

In the process of assisting an individual in finding the right solution for their problem, situation or goal, this advisor would need to perform four major tasks: (i) listening to the needs of the end user and translate those into a search strategy that complements the digital advisory component; (ii) identifying relevant solutions and suppliers, and assess their pertinence towards each situation; (iii) assisting and guiding the individual during the decision-making process; and (iv) following up on satisfaction and stimulating users to provide feedback on the platform [42].

There are several groups that are in need of advice and consultancy on AAL solutions and thus could benefit from the existence of the Authorised Active Advisors. In accordance with previous classifications of AAL stakeholders [32], the following stakeholder groups have been identified within the ActiveAdvice project as the main beneficiaries: (i) older adults (primary stakeholders); and (ii) professional and informal caregivers (secondary stakeholders) [26, 43].

As stressed above, older adults are still facing many difficulties when it comes to technology use. Moreover, AAL solutions require close monitoring as those usually deliver crucial services that might have a transformative benefit in older adults lives [3]. Indeed, as Wild and colleagues [44] reported, it is the lack of knowledge of how ICT services can increase or support autonomy that prevents older adults from using them. Until such technologies are seen as personally relevant and useful to their lives, older adults might be reluctant to accept them or learn the necessary skills to operate them. The challenge is, therefore, to understand each persons individual situation and provide guidance in the process of finding the most suitable AAL solution.

In addition to older adults, informal and professional caregivers play a vital role in the decision-making process. They often have a supportive or influential role regarding care decisions, as the former provide the older adults with unpaid and ongoing assistance with basic or instrumental activities of daily living; the latter offer specialized services to the care receiver and are trained and qualified individuals. Furthermore, some AAL solutions explicitly target this group rather than older adults themselves, e.g. in supporting care or monitoring of health conditions or behaviours [5]. Similar to older adults, informal and professional caregivers possess heterogeneous competencies, interests, and needs both regarding care provision and ICT use to this end. Moreover, regarding professional caregivers, an important aspect that negatively influences the uptake or prescription of AAL solutions by professional caregivers is the lack of proper training and guidance when new technologies are introduced into the care process and thus they can be reluctant in accepting such technologies [44].

3 Methodology

Based on a multi-stakeholder perspective, a comprehensive literature review together with a qualitative study were conducted to identify the prospective benefits of AAL advisors, their profile, and required knowledge and skills to perform this role. Outcomes from this study were used to refine the concept of Authorised Active Advisors and to develop a training outline based on an explorative analysis of their needs, competencies and requirements (see Fig. 1).

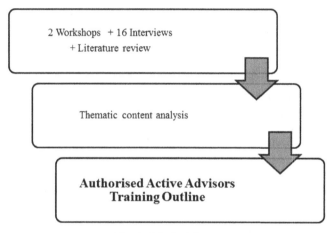

Fig. 1. Methodology.

3.1 Literature Review

A literature search of scientific publications on a selection of databases was conducted, aimed at identifying experiences and practices (if available) on education and profes-sional specialization for AAL advisors. First, a list of keywords was compiled: the term Ambient Assisted Living was kept fixed and combined alternatively with eight additional terms defined on the basis of the previous literature exploration. Table 1 presents the databases selected, keywords used, the number of hits per search given, and the number of selected articles for analysis after the removal of duplications and the exclusion of irrelevant papers (for example, papers within the general topic of AAL which discussed learning or training from a computer science perspective; focus on AAL technologies as training devices themselves, etc. – in short, any paper that contained the selected keywords but was a mismatch for the scope of the literature analysis).

    Papers found using more than one keyword combination are reported just once in Table 1. Selected papers were fully read, and subjected to a thematic content analysis and an interpretive qualitative synthesis of the main themes emerging from the selected literature was performed (see Sect. 4). Insights arising from the literature search are neither exhaustive nor are they representative, as an explorative approach was chosen given the nature of the knowledge we aimed to produce, i.e. a comprehensive literature search was chosen over a systematic one because a broad question – experiences and practices – was posed to be explored.

3.2 Primary Data Collection and Analysis

Two workshops with a total of 14 participants and semi-structured interviews with 16 different stakeholders that potentially fit the human advisor profile were conducted (e.g., formal caregivers, council workers, people working on organizations that advocate for older adults, etc.). The two workshops took place at the AAL Forum 2018 in Bilbao, Spain (n = 9) and in the Netherlands (n = 5). While the workshop at the AAL Forum involved members of the AAL community, from different European countries and with diverse backgrounds (e.g. social sciences, engineering), the workshop in the Netherlands involved employees of the municipality of Alkmaar, who already provided advisory services to older adults and their relatives or informal caregivers on health and care-related issues/resources.

The interviews were carried out in five different countries: Austria, Belgium, the Netherlands, Portugal, and the UK. A single interview schedule was designed by the research team and properly translated to be used in each partner country. The contents from the workshops and interviews were transcribed and subjected to a thematic content analysis. All contents were coded according to three main themes, defined deductively: Benefits and profile of the Authorised Active Advisors; Skills and Knowledge of the Authorised Active Advisors; and Preferences on the training concept for Authorised Active Advisors. Sub-themes emerged inductively from the analysis.

4 Results and Discussion

As a result of the analysis, we were able to gather some valuable insights regarding (i) training for advisors on AAL solutions, including existing initiatives and practices (see Sect. 4.1. Literature review outcomes); (ii) prospective benefits, profile, skills and knowledge, and preferences on the training concept for Authorised Active Advisors (see Sect. 4.2. Lessons learned from interviews and collaborative workshops). Based on the insights gathered, a training concept is outlined as a final output (see Sect. 5).

4.1 Literature Insights: Education for Ambient Assisted Living Technologies and Services

Overall, 42 papers were selected taking into consideration the relevance of their title and abstract (see Table 1). They were then analysed and subjected to a thematic content analysis. After further and more detailed analysis, only very few papers were considered for this research, unveiling a gap in research with regards to training for AAL advisory services.

Table 1. Search history for selected scientific publications.

Keywords (AND,)	Database	Hits (Selected)
Training needs AND Ambient Assisted Living	Scopus	20 (3)
	SAGE	10 (1)
	Web of Science	6 (1)
	PubMed	5 (1)
	EBSCO	1 (0)
Professions AND Ambient Assisted Living	Scopus	3 (2)
	SAGE	4 (1)
	Web of Science	0
	PubMed	1 (1)
	EBSCO	0
Education AND Ambient Assisted Living	Scopus	49 (3)
	SAGE	28 (3)
	Web of Science	8 (2)
	PubMed	15 (4)
	EBSCO	10 (1)
Training AND Ambient Assisted Living	Scopus	91 (0)
	SAGE	6 (0)
	Web of Science	37 (0)
	PubMed	21 (4)
	EBSCO	14 (1)
Jobs AND Ambient Assisted Living	Scopus	18 (1)
	SAGE	4 (0)
	Web of Science	2 (0)

(*continued*)

Table 1. (*continued*)

	PubMed	0 (0)
	EBSCO	1 (0)
Skills AND Ambient Assisted Living	Scopus	39 (2)
	SAGE	24 (1)
	Web of Science	8 (0)
	PubMed	3 (1)
	EBSCO	9 (1)
Learning AND Ambient Assisted Living	Scopus	298 (0)
	SAGE	35 (0)
	Web of Science	103 (3)
	PubMed	27 (2)
	EBSCO	39(0)
Knowledge AND Ambient Assisted Living	Scopus	273 (0)
	SAGE	42 (0)
	Web of Science	71 (0)
	PubMed	22 (1)
	EBSCO	30 (2)

The analysis, aiming to identify patterns and themes within the selected publications, resulted in the aggregation of contents within the identified topics, which are synthesized below (see Sects. 4.1, 4.2, 4.3 and 4.4).

Overall, one can conclude from this review that acceptance of AAL is rising and its implementation is becoming a rapidly growing economic sector where new jobs are created. However, proper education for qualifying employees in the AAL area is still massively lagging behind [20, 36]. The lack of education and training may be a major impediment in the successful adoption of AAL solutions [29]. Thus, as highlighted by Illiger and colleagues [22], it is necessary that care workers, health service professionals as well as technicians and craftsmen in the field obtain continuous training to become capable consultants/advisors for AAL solutions. A few training experiences for AAL consultancy experiences are documented in the literature, those being explored in the next sections.

Target Groups: Who is Trained to Offer Advice? Several target groups are mentioned in the literature, with most publications high-lighting the relevance of training heterogeneous groups [6, 7, 9, 33]. While Bruder and colleagues [9] designed a training course for managers in health care, caregivers, managers in the housing industry, decision makers, engineers, developers and other technical staff who are also involved in the development and distribution of AAL products. Behrends and colleagues [6] targeted health professionals, crafts-men and technicians. Behrends et al. [7] and Nitschke et al. [33] focused on health professions, craftsmen and individuals with a background in engineering or similar areas. Barakat et al. [5] see healthcare professionals, including nurses, professions allied with medicine, social workers, healthcare managers, and caregivers as the core target group to make the best use of technology within a care context. Keijzer-Broers and de Reuver [24], on the other hand, see a special potential for installers to bridge the gap between technology and end users (in particular, for smart homes) due to their existing relationship with them. They have a combined knowledge of the demand and daily living of end users as well as of the technology. However, they do have limited knowledge of smart living, lack commercial and marketing skills, and focus on technology rather than user experience [24]. Katzmaier [23] refers that the implementation of age-related case management, a figure ensuring counselling with respect to AAL, is requested. The INVERSIA project allows designing recommendations for an AAL-Case Management, showing that relatives and social service providers are considered fundamental target groups in the consultation process.

Overall, those experiences were concerned in enrolling qualified individuals with backgrounds mostly on health-related and technology-related fields but also care-givers of people in need of AAL solutions.

Necessary Knowledge, Skills and Competencies: What Does an AAL Advisor Need to Know? There is a need to establish the multiple skills and competencies which are required for being able to provide advice on AAL solutions. This, of course, depends on the target group in question. For example, teaching technical aspects to trainees without a technical background (e.g. healthcare professionals) is necessary but can be challenging [9, 44].

In a study developed by Barakat and her colleagues [5], they identified and organized the set of skills and competencies of healthcare professionals in five areas:

– requirements for basic ICT skills for using technology and hardware, proficiency, quantitative analysis, and interpretation skills,
– communication skills,
– support and guidance for the patient (both for care support, computer, and ICT use),
– knowledge of best practices, and
– legal requirements concerning patient privacy and confidentiality.

The engAGEnt project [14], which aimed to develop and test a harmonized European curriculum based on ECVET principles of what will qualify people for the job role of an AAL Specialist or Consultant, identified the need to analyse the living situation of an older person to identify suitable AAL solutions for their individual case. For this, they need (i) knowledge of new, digital technologies in order to identify and manage technological solutions, and (ii) awareness of relevant care and support requirements of the individuals [14].

Bruder et al. [9] analysed the educational demands of the target group. Main results stressed the need:

– for an overview of currently available AAL solutions;
– of R&D in this field;
– of the functionality of assistive technology and its benefits;
– of how to plan, implement and finance complex AAL systems;
– of the presentation, classification, and evaluation of systems regarding ethical aspects;
– of declarations and general legal conditions;
– to exchange experiences with other professionals.

Based on this, Bruder et al. [9] defined a set of educational objectives. In this sense, participants should be:

– able to plan and accompany the design and implementation of a complex AAL system for a specific demand – this includes knowing which kind of products are currently in the market and which ideas are under research and judging on with technology is appropriate for a certain demand;
– able to understand the general technical functionality and the social dimension of an AAL system;
– aware of ethical and legal aspects related to AAL systems;
– able to find and discuss AAL solutions in interdisciplinary teams.

In turn, according to Behrends et al. [6] knowledge on the following topics is required:

– demographic change;
– the characteristics of the AAL target group; technological basics;
– funding opportunities; and
– critical aspects and consulting training.

For Heuner, Loeffler and Schmidt [20] the topics covered must be related to advisory skills; law and financing; disease patterns and needs of the elderly; housing; ethical aspects; and systems for AAL.

Gomersal et al. [18] outlined an evaluation concept for AAL solutions which provides useful synergies for AAL trainings: the key question is to understand what works, for whom, in what context. Any technological support needs to respond to a unique combination of psychosocial and occupational needs of each person [18] and an advisor on AAL solutions should then be able to understand, evaluate and select AAL solutions based on these aspects. Gomersal et al. [18] also suggest evaluations that go beyond the individual level and take into account the whole network to understand how technology produces effects, and what kind of networks are needed for the technology to be beneficial to a person.

Nitschke and colleagues [33] highlighted the following needed competencies:

- knowledge of AAL (professional expertise/competence);
- communication skills (social competence);
- problem-solving ability (method competence); and
- personal ability to reflect (personal competence).

Regarding the consultation situation, the conclusions from Katzmaiers study [23] shows that the closest possible orientation towards the needs of the clients is considered a fundamental success factor. An independent consultation without pressure to sell is also appreciated, as well as solutions which offer the best possible fulfilment of needs and are as cost-efficient as possible.

To summarise, the following skills are key for any education focussing on AAL technologies:

- basic understanding of (using) ICT, and functionality of relevant technologies including the social dimension of an AAL system;
- an overview of the AAL market, currently available AAL solutions and other assistive technologies, and main R&D projects in this area;
- legal requirements and ethical standards, including privacy and confidentiality spects issues;
- financing of AAL solutions;
- communication skills and social competence;
- multidisciplinary working skills;
- awareness of the individual context of AAL advisory beneficiaries, of the ageing process and demographic trends.

Training Approaches and Concepts: What is the Best Way of Training? In order for professionals to develop the required competencies, adequate training concepts and approaches need to be defined. An explicit reference to the training course conceptual approach was not given in most of the analysed papers. However, Bruder and colleagues [9], state to have adopted a student centered training concept as well as approached the AAL concept from a sociotechnical perspective, which combines technical systems, social contact and service to support elderly people in their daily life at home.

In turn, learning/teaching methods used to train AAL advisors are more frequently described when characterizing the training courses. The most popular included: (i) the use of everyday, realistic scenarios and example cases to illustrate and role play advisory situations (e.g., [6, 9, 33]); (ii) the offer of hands-on experiences including demonstration/experimentation of AAL technologies by the advisor, for instance resorting to living labs (e.g., [6, 9]); (iii) self-learning/study resorting to physical resources (e.g., [9]; (iv) self-learning/study resorting to digital platforms/tools (e.g., [20]); and (v) traditional classroom seminars/lectures [6, 9, 20]. Behrends and colleagues [6], when asking the participants of a training module pilot to rate the usefulness of different learning/teaching methods, found that case examples were the most preferred method. According to Nitschke et al. [33], a suitable approach is the use of everyday scenarios and example cases with theoretical inputs about the context, the subjective experience of the user, etc. This allows training participants to learn how to make a decision within a particular scenario, which needs to be as realistic as possible. The EngAGEnt project also highlights the importance of having a scenario-based approach, which means that the knowledge, skills, and competences to be achieved at the end of the training are to be acquired against a backdrop of a real-life scenario [14]. Regarding the training modality, most initiatives report having adopted a blended learning approach (e.g., [6, 7, 20]). A blended learning approach was pointed out as the most suitable training approach, combining online (e-learning) with f2f learning methodologies [7]. Technology-enabled learning can play a vital role in contemporary education structures [40]. Therefore, blended learning is an effective approach and creates a rich educational environment since it increases learning outside the traditional f2f learning environment and has a positive impact on student motivation and performance in general [17, 21]. Heussner and colleagues [20], for instance, resorted to an online platform integrating an information tool, a serious game and a forum, allowing for self-learning and information exchange.

Concerning the training course structure (i.e. number of hours, modules), it largely varied across different training experiences. For instance, while the course described by Heuner and colleagues [20] consisted of three seminar days with a two month self-study period in between, other courses where more time demanding (e.g., 40 lessons each module in Behrends et al. [6]), and organized in several modules (e.g., [6, 9]).

Challenges and Ethical Considerations: What Does an AAL Advisor Need to Take into Account? There are some challenges regarding the design of training courses for AAL advisory. Behrends and colleagues [6] identify three main challenges: first, AAL technologies are very diverse and can range from stand-alone assistive devices to fully integrated smart homes; and they can contemplate a range of areas such as health & care; safety & security; information & communication; among others. Yet, in spite of their broader coverage, AAL solutions are still largely underrepresented in the market which hampers the job of the AAL advisor. Second, AAL solutions must be adapted to the needs of the users and this requires a comprehensive view of the users, considering their needs and contexts. Third, provision of good advice regarding AAL solutions most likely requires the collaboration between different professional groups, usually having their own professional cultures and languages. In addition, Bruder and colleagues [9] stressed the challenge of teaching technical aspects to trainees without a technical background.

Furthermore, there are ethical considerations that need to be taken into account. When giving advice, especially to vulnerable people, as for instance persons with a cognitive limitation (e.g. dementia), they might lack the capacity to decide for themselves whether to make use of a particular technology. Moreover, privacy and security issues are of relevance considering, for instance, the amount of personal and sometimes sensitive data existing in the cloud when using AAL solutions, frequently interchanged with a large number of devices always connected [16]. As stressed by Bruder and colleagues [9] privacy awareness is an absolute necessity for AAL advisors. Therefore, certain factors have to be considered on an individual level such as the persons past and present concerns and perspectives and the benefits that might be achieved by using technology [25].

4.2   Lessons Learned from Interviews and Collaborative Workshops

From the interviews and collaborative workshops analysis, it was possible to identify three main themes: Benefits and profile of the Authorised Active Advisors; Skills and Knowledge of the Authorised Active Advisors; and Preferences on the training concept for Authorised Active Advisors. The lessons learned in each theme are presented in the following subsections.

Benefits and Profile of the Authorised Active Advisors. The value proposition of the Authorised Active Advisor contemplates benefits for all three target groups of the ActiveAdvice digital decision-support platform [43]. Older adults, as well as their relatives, have shown a preference to receive advice personally. This f2f contact is seen as a facilitator of personalisation, which constitutes a major benefit since it gives a response to the users needs. Moreover, it is perceived as a contribution to prevent social isolation by establishing human interaction, which consequently has a major impact in gaining the users trust, as previously described [11, 34, 35, 41, 43]. Therefore, the primary stakeholders – older adults [26, 43] – directly benefit from the Authorised Active Advisor, whose activities should consist of assisting older adults to access AAL content, helping them to choose and buy products and services, recommending technology that will support them and providing comprehensive information and knowledge on AAL solutions. The Authorised Active Advisor could guarantee that there is a proper response to the consumer's real needs, articulating those with the right product or solution and avoiding, at the same time, an information overload that could be harmful to the decision process. Although Authorised Active Advisors would primarily play an advisory role towards older adults (and informal and professional caregivers), businesses and governments might also benefit from them. The lack of general public awareness of AAL technologies and their potential benefits are identified by business stakeholders as an obstacle to introduce and succeed with these products and services in the market, a challenge that can be overcome by Authorised Active Advisors. Moreover, reducing stigmatization of AAL technologies, promoting market equipment attractively and offering differentiation over other catalogue websites (that do not contemplate a human advisor component) are some of the foreseen positive impacts on businesses. For governments, the existence of the Authorised Active Advisor has the potential to increase the number of people self-funding AAL solutions and, on the other hand, to reduce the number of people using council services (e.g. care institutions).

As one of the key concepts of the ActiveAdvice project, a clear definition of the intended profile of Authorised Active Advisors is needed. From the participants perspectives, we conceptualised two advisor profiles: the Authorised Active Advisor either (i) works in an existing organisation or a business within the ageing and care market (AAL product development, care advisory to older adults, sales and marketing, social care organisations, education) (profile A) or (ii) has practical care/medical experience and know-how in dealing with older people (i.e. gerontologists, occupational therapists, social educators, etc.) (profile B) (see Fig. 2). The importance of having someone with (professional) experience in the ageing field was stressed by participants and is in accordance with the possibilities previously considered by the consortium.

Figure 2 illustrates the two profiles of the Authorised Active Advisors as well as the different target groups for AAL advisory services. Since the appropriate support is offered on an individual basis, there is no distinction made between the human advisor profiles and advisees – older adults, informal and professional caregivers (see Fig. 2 above). Nonetheless, further research is necessary to study whether and how the different Authorised Active Advisor profiles have an impact on the way the different target groups/advisees are advised. The content and context are needed to be taken into consideration. In addition, it is also important to further understand the relationship of the quality of the individual advisory in context to the two profiles. This would also provide important feedback on the training programme.

Skills and Knowledge of the Authorised Active Advisors. From the data collection, it was also possible to identify a set of skills and knowledge that Authorised Active

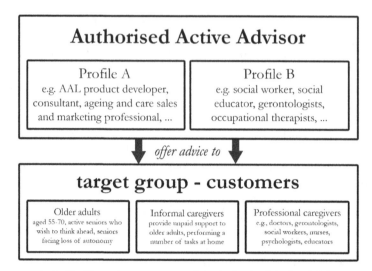

Fig. 2. Profile and target groups of the Authorised Active Advisor.

Advisors should have. In this sense, there are two key areas in which Authorised Active Advisors must demonstrate knowledge and skills: (i) social skills, and (ii) knowledge about ICT, technology in general and AAL. It must be noted, here, that interpersonal relationship skills like empathy, patience, communication, trust were considered to be more important prerequisites than technical knowledge.

Besides the two main areas mentioned above, it was also pointed out that Authorised Active Advisors should have a general understanding of the ageing process and its different challenges, namely having some general knowledge regarding main diseases or health problems associated with the ageing process, such as dementia. Also, they should have some knowledge about the difficulties underlying people's lives – for example, know or have some information about the context where the person lives, their health conditions, what they need was highlighted. Furthermore, as Authorised Active Advisors will also be resorting to the ActiveAdvice platform, some general knowledge regarding the ActiveAdvice project is mandatory, namely what the core values, vision and mission of the ActiveAdvice are. Lastly, Authorised Active Advisors need to have a certain flair, social commitment and intrinsic motivation to offer advice and assist older adults in their local community. Indeed, the participants considered that the advisors should work on a regional/local level, since knowing very well the local context where the person in need for advice is inserted is fundamental to properly recommend local resources and inform about existing financial incentives and measures (e.g., reimbursement possibilities), which is, in turn, another important area of knowledge to promote.

Lifelong learning implies the idea that knowledge can be acquired and skills can be developed anywhere and anytime, so despite the existing knowledge and skills as well as professional and personal experiences that potential Authorised Active Advisors already have, it is necessary to provide further training. To follow the same training programme is also crucial in order to guarantee some coherence and homogenization regarding the profile: this way, an adequate training levels out the differences between the two profiles, ensuring that people with different backgrounds are able to gain the same level of knowledge and skills necessary to act as an Authorised Active Advisor.

Preferences on the Training Concept for Authorised Active Advisors. The content of a specific training course depends, among other factors, on the attributes, needs and prior knowledge of the target group. It also depends on the way the course is delivered. The participants showed a clear preference for a blended approach, where both online and f2f sessions are available, which is aligned with the literature found at this respect and previously discussed.

For the online component, learning/teaching methods suggested by the participants include having educational material available online, and the organization of webinars were also mentioned. For the f2f sessions, participants suggested group sessions and the handing of educational material for self-study. Practical exercises/role-playing resorting to the ActiveAdvice platform and hands-on experiences for testing and evaluating AAL products were also highlighted as preferred strategies to use.

As outlined above, there are diverse groups of stakeholders targeted to provide consultancy and advice on AAL. The heterogeneity of the mentioned groups (see e.g., [6, 7, 9, 33]) can be a strength for a training approach. While cooperation, especially with organisations from other sectors, is a challenge, it also has distinct benefits, especially in sharing knowledge in a bottom-up way [24].

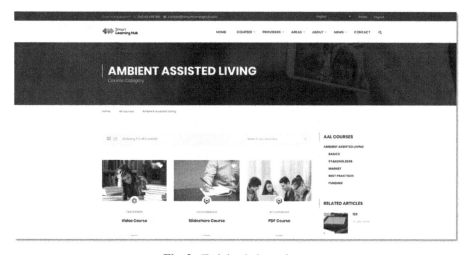

Fig. 3. Training hub mock-up.

Named as an explicit educational objective by Bruder and colleagues [9], AAL solutions should be discussed in interdisciplinary teams. Interdisciplinary cooperation is, then, especially important for AAL since the implementation of technology-based health services for older people always requires that different professional groups work together ([7]; see also Behrends et al. [7]). In this sense, the academic and/or professional background can be different.

5   Training Concept Outline

Considering the Authorised Active Advisor profile, as well as their skills and knowledge which is seen as mandatory by the interviewees and workshop participants, a training concept was developed as an output of this study. As educational objectives, at the end of the course, trainees must be able to: (i) identify AAL solutions and suppliers and assess their pertinence towards users needs, resorting to the ActiveAdvice platform; (ii) translate users needs into a search strategy; (iii) assist and guide the individual during the decision-making process; (iv) create, collect and/or resort to real-life testimonies, comments and ratings of products and services; and (v) refer users to the correct authorities/advisors in regards to questions on reimbursement, assessment, complaints or others. From the data analysis, we conceptualize a course outline based on a blended learning approach where the future Authorised Active Advisors could benefit from digital and f2f training sessions. F2f sessions allow trainees to exchange experiences and doubts, deepen their knowledge and be involved in role-play activities. In turn, online sessions, where trainees will be able to access theoretical contents, were considered by the study participants as an effective approach to achieving full proficiency. Another positive aspect of using a blended learning approach is that it can accommodate an increasingly diverse student population whilst adding value to the learning environment through the incorporation of online teaching resources [2]. It offers students the chance of managing part of the learning process based on each persons timetable – everyone can connect from anywhere to receive online training [19].

Based on findings from both the literature analysis and qualitative study, and taking into account a preference for a blended-learning training modality, a mock-up for a training hub was designed within the ActiveAdvice project (see Fig. 3).

This mock-up/platform (see Fig. 3) has been developed primarily for workers f organisations or businesses within the ageing and care market (Profile A) or workers with practical care or medical experience and know-how in dealing with older people (Profile B), who would be interested in expanding their knowledge and broaden their job opportunities.

Regarding the training programme content, and according to insights gathered in the research carried, the course is organized into five modules: (i) the ActiveAdvice project and the digital ActiveAdvice decision-support platform; (ii) Ageing Process; (iii) Ambient Assisted Living Technologies; (iv) Reimbursement and Administration; and (v) Communication and Human Relation. It is important to highlight that the national context and its particularities will be taken into account when designing each module (e.g. for funding and reimbursement issues).

Part of module 3, Ambient Assisted Living Technologies, is information about the TAALXONOMY [28], a use-case based classification system for AAL solutions. The TAALXONOMY consists of eight main use cases (scopes of application) and 43 scenarios (areas of application). Knowledge about this classification system is also necessary to understand the logic of the ActiveAdvice platform, which follows the TAALXONOMYs use-case based approach.

Considering the main objectives of the training as well as its programme, a set of learning outcomes were delineated in accordance (Fig. 4).

Modules	Programme	Learning outcomes
1. ActiveAdvice Project & Decision-support Platform	1.1..Introduction to the Active-Advice project: 1.1.1 ActiveAdvice contextu-alization 1.1.2.Aims and principles 1.2. Introduction to ActiveAdvice platform & its usage 1.3. ActiveAdvice code of con-duct	The learner knows the objectives of the ActiveAdvice project and what is expected from them as Authorised Active Advisors; The learner knows how to use the Active-Advice platform and be able to assist others in using it; The learner knows and is able to follow the code of conduct.
2.Ageing Process	2.1. Physical, Cognitive and Social Impacts of Ageing 2.1.1. Health-related prob-lems 2.1.2. Social impacts of age-ing 2.2.. Older adults and ICT	The learner has general knowledge regard-ing the ageing process and its impacts; The learner has general knowledge regard-ing the most frequent age-related conditions (dementia, Parkinson, Alzheimer's, etc.) and the possibilities to use technological solutions;
3.Ambient Assisted Living (AAL) technologies	3.1. AAL overview & core tech-nologies 3.2. Benefits and Challenges of AAL 3.2.1. TAALXONOMY classification model 3.2.2. Existing AAL products and services 3.3.. Future market developments 3.4.. Interoperability	The learner has a broad knowledge of AAL technologies: classification and types; The learner is able to identify the challenges and constraints and explain the benefits of using AAL solutions; The learner is able to give advice by corre-lating the user needs with the different AAL products and solutions available; The learner knows the basics of businesses relevant to AAL; The learner knows which solutions are compatible, and has a basic knowledge of the quality standards used in AAL technol-ogies.
4.Reimbursement and administration	4.1. Reimbursement policies and practices - the local reality 4.2. Legal requirements & frameworks	The learner knows the essential reimburse-ment policies of their local context; The learner is familiar with the country-specific legal framework relevant to work with AAL; The learner knows relevant local resources and initiatives related to AAL (e.g. funded projects); The learner knows where to find necessary and essential additional information on this topic.
5.Communication and Human Rela-tions	5.1..Communicability and com-munication modes 5.1.1. Customer Service Skills 5.2.Interpersonal relations - integral and humanized 5.2.1.Decision-making and cooperation 5.2.2. Active Listening & Empathy	The learner demonstrates interpersonal skills to ensure confidence and trust; The learner is able to actively listening and show empathy and patience; The learner shows communication skills and strategies to engage users in the deci-sion-making process.

Fig. 4. Training Course outline.

6 Conclusion

Previous work from the ActiveAdvice project shows that end users are willing to learn which products or services are useful for their specific situation, what makes their life easier or where and how to find a specific product [43]. The ActiveAdvice platform provides the much-needed information on AAL products and services, thus helping the users to gather detailed insights before buying a product or asking for a service. Advice is considered a key service that can have a great impact on and bring significant benefits to people who resort to this kind of digital platforms. In this sense, having a human advisory component in addition to the purely digital platform could have a great impact on the way users resort to the ActiveAdvice platform. Authorised Active Advisors are able to fill a gap in the decision-making process that an otherwise exclusively digital environment cannot fill, due to the possibility for personal contact and human interaction, and contextual knowledge for the individual situation. The integrated service logic connected to the concept of Authorised Active Advisors may allow personalisation of feedback, increased trust of end users as well as higher-quality advice.

According to a previous study carried out within the ActiveAdvice project [8, 42], an Authorised Active Advisor can be conceptualized as a mediator between AAL providers and end users, helping the end users with the process of making informed decisions. They are a human touch to the digital platform.

Hence, we can recognize the added value of Authorised Active Advisors in several aspects: (i) personal contact and human touch; (ii) trust; (iii) context knowledge; (iv) ability to fill gaps in the digital advisor system; (v) confidence and autonomy; and (vi) decision support.

The ActiveAdvice technical solution offers the tools and the digital intelligence to the Authorised Active Advisors, so they can provide end users with up-to-date, useful and applicable knowledge about AAL products and services, options for financial support and customer feedback. The advisory process can be quite complex and result in very specific questions, sometimes only answered by specialists in a particular domain. Therefore, Authorised Active Advisors can benefit from the European scope of the ActiveAdvice platform and the connection with other registered advisors. Furthermore, advice in AAL needs a multidisciplinary approach, taking into account different areas of expertise (from general knowledge about the ageing process to ICT and e.g. questions of interoperability to questions of reimbursement and the national legislation, as outlined above) and different professional backgrounds [6, 7].

The idea of developing a community of Authorised Active Advisors can work as a good opportunity, allowing different advisors to share experiences, specific knowledge, and general expertise on different topics. In order to develop such a community, it is important to explore the possibilities of different channels of communication. It is important to note that online channels are of a distinct benefit for the scope of ActiveAdvice, as they (i) allow advisors to exchange knowledge and expertise across geographical borders, and (ii) can allow a time independent knowledge exchange.

However, many open questions remain regarding the human advisor concept. First, trust in the advisor is a core question requirement interviews carried out within the project [43] showed that a concern is around the neutrality vs. expertise of the advisor (for instance business actors perceived advice as being best given by those who sell a product, who are, on the other hand, not neutral actors). Second, growing old and being in need of care is a rather local experience, therefore different advisor profiles are probable to emerge in distinct local realities. It is up to the ActiveAdvice project to come up with a detailed training concept to provide the necessary knowledge and leverage the full potential of the integrated service logic.

References

1. AAL-Programme: Strategy 2014–2020 for the active and assisted living programme (2014). http://www.aal-europe.eu/wpcontent/uploads/2015/11/20151001-AAL-Strategy-Final.pdf
2. Alammary, A., Sheard, J., Carbone, A.: Blended learning in higher education: three different design approaches. Australas. J. Educ. Technol. **30**(4) (2014)
3. Alsulami, M.H., Atkins, A.S., Campion, R.J.: Factors influencing the adoption of ambient assisted living technologies by healthcare providers in the Kingdom of Saudi Arabia. In: Ezziyyani, M., Bahaj, M., Khoukhi, F. (eds.) AIT2S 2017. LNNS, vol. 25, pp. 3–11. Springer, Cham (2018). https://doi.org/10.1007/978-3-319-69137-4_1
4. Baldissera, T.A., Camarinha-Matos, L.M.: Towards a collaborative business ecosystem for elderly care. In: Camarinha-Matos, L.M., Falcão, A.J., Vafaei, N., Najdi, S. (eds.) DoCEIS 2016. IAICT, vol. 470, pp. 24–34. Springer, Cham (2016). https://doi.org/10.1007/978-3-319-31165-4_3
5. Barakat, A., Woolrych, R.D., Sixsmith, A., Kearns, W.D., Kort, H.S.: ehealth technology competencies for health professionals working in home care to support older adults to age in place: outcomes of a two-day collaborative workshop. Medicine 2.0 **2**(2) (2013)
6. Behrends, M., et al.: A certified qualification course for aal consultants for health professionals and services, craftsmen and technicians-design, results and perspectives. Biomed. Tech. **59**, 418–421 (2014)
7. Behrends, M., Stiller, G., Illiger, K., Nitschke, M., Egbert, N., Krückeberg, J.: E-learning as integral part of teaching-learning processes in continuing education for ambient assisted living technologies and services. Biomed. Eng./Biomedizinische Technik (2013)
8. Bertel, D., et al.: High tech, high touch: integrating digital and human aal advisory services for older adults. In: ICT4AWE 2018, Funchal, Portugal, 22–23 March 2018, vol. 1, pp. 241–249. SciTePress-Science and Technology Publications (2018)
9. Bruder, I., Heuer, A., Karopka, T., Schuldt, J., Kosche, K.: Experiences in developing and testing an ambient assisted living course for further education. In: Yin, X., Ho, K., Zeng, D., Aickelin, U., Zhou, R., Wang, H. (eds.) HIS 2015. LNCS, vol. 9085. pp. 154–164. Springer, Heidelberg (2015)
10. Cummins, S., Peltier, J.W., A. Schibrowsky, J., Nill, A.: Consumer behavior in the online context. J. Res. Interact. Market. **8**(3), 169–202 (2014)
11. Damodaran, L., Olphert, W.: User responses to assisted living technologies: a review of the literature. J. Integr. Care **18**(2), 25–32 (2010). https://doi.org/10.5042/jic.2010.0133
12. Denis, A.: Human advisor workflow. D3.4, ActiveAdvice AAL Programme Project No. 851908 (2017)
13. Doyle, J., Bailey, C., Scanaill, C.N., van den Berg, F.: Lessons learned in deploying independent living technologies to older adults homes. Univ. Access Inf. Soc. **13**(2), 191–204 (2014)
14. engAGEnt: Aal consultant training curriculum. background, guidelines and documents for the qualification as aal consultant. 2012-1-DE2-LEO05-11223 (2014)
15. Breidbach, C.F., Brodie, R., Hollebeek, L.: Beyond virtuality: from engagement platforms to engagement ecosystems. Manag. Serv. Qual. **24**(6), 592–611 (2014). https://doi.org/10.1108/MSQ-08-2013-0158

16. Ferreira, A., Teles, S., Vieira-Marques, P.: Sotraace for smart security in ambient assisted living. J. Ambient Intell. Smart Environ. **11**(4), 323–334 (2019)
17. Geng, S., Law, K.M.Y., Niu, B.: Investigating self-directed learning and technology readiness in blending learning environment. Int. J. Educ. Technol. High. Educ. **16**(1), 1–22 (2019). https://doi.org/10.1186/s41239-019-0147-0
18. Gomersall, T., et al.: Network-based approaches for evaluating ambient assisted living (AAL) technologies. Evaluation **23**(2), 192–208 (2017)
19. Herrador-Alcaide, T.C., Hernández-Solís, M., Galván, R.S.: Feelings of satisfaction in mature students of financial accounting in a virtual learning environment: an experience of measurement in higher education. Int. J. Educ. Technol. High. Educ. **16**(1), 20 (2019)
20. Heussner, M., Loeffler, B., Schmidt, L.: Design and evaluation of a further education for persons working in aal context. Biomed. Eng. Biomedizinische Technik **59**, S447–S450 (2014)
21. Ibrahim, M.M., Nat, M.: Blended learning motivation model for instructors in higher education institutions. Int. J. Educ. Technol. High. Educ. **16**(1), 1–21 (2019). https://doi.org/10.1186/s41239-019-0145-2
22. Illiger, K., et al.: Transferring learning to practice with e-learning-experiences in continuing education in the field of ambient assisted living. In: eHealth, pp. 180–187 (2014)
23. Katzmaier, S.: Ambient assisted living-design recommendations for a case management and a respective business model. Int. J. Integr. Care **16**(6) (2016)
24. Keijzer-Broers, W., de Reuver, M.: Cooperation and knowledge challenges in realizing smart homes: the case of small installer businesses. Indoor Built Environ. **27**(2), 184–193 (2018)
25. Kenigsberg, P.A., et al.: Assistive technologies to address capabilities of people with dementia: from research to practice. Dementia **18**(4), 1568–1595 (2019)
26. Kofler, A.C., Schmitter, P.: User requirements, decision workflow and use cases report. D2.3, ActiveAdvice AAL Programme Project No. 851908 (2017)
27. Kofler, A.Ch., A.S.G., Schmitter, P.: Baseline report on AAL advice, decision and authorization. D2.1, ActiveAdvice AAL Programme Project No. 851908 (2016)
28. Leitner, P., Neuschmid, J., Ruscher, S.: Taalxonomy: Entwicklung einer praktikablen axonomie zur effektiven klassifizierung von aal-produkten und dienstleistungen. Studienbericht im Rahmen des Technologieprogramm benefit. Wien (2015)
29. Mantzana, V., Themistocleous, M., Morabito, V.: Healthcare information systems and older employees' training. J. Enterprise Inf. Manag. **23**(6), 680–693 (2010)
30. Marschollek, M., Mix, S., Wolf, K.H., Effertz, B., Haux, R., Steinhagen-Thiessen, E.: Ict-based health information services for elderly people: past experiences, current trends, and future strategies. Med. Inform. Internet Med. **32**(4), 251–261 (2007)
31. Michel, J.P., Franco, A.: Geriatricians and technology. J. Am. Med. Directors Assoc. **15**(12), 860–862 (2014)
32. Nedopil, C., Schauber, C., Glende, I.: Aal stakeholders and their requirement. Report by the Ambient and Assisted Living Association (2013)
33. Nitschke, M., Krckeberg, J., Egbert, N., Schmeer, R., Mascia, M., Goll, S.: Entwicklung und durchfhrung einer interprofessionellen qualifizierungsmanahme zum aal-berater. erfahrungen, ergebnisse und lessons learned einer beruflichen weiterbildung fr gesundheitsberufe, handwerk und technik im projekt mhh-quaal. Pdagogik der Gesundheitsberufe - Die Zeitschrift fr den interprofessionellen Dialog 1, pp. 15–23 (2014)
34. Novitzky, P., et al.: A review of contemporary work on the ethics of ambient assisted living technologies for people with Dementia. Sci. Eng. Ethics **21**(3), 707–765 (2014). https://doi.org/10.1007/s11948-014-9552-x
35. Olphert, W., Damodaran, L., Balatsoukas, P., Parkinson, C.: Process requirements for building sustainable digital assistive technology for older people. J. Assist. Technol. **3**(3), 4–13 (2009)

36. Panagiotakopoulos, T., Theodosiou, A., Kameas, A.: Exploring ambient assisted living job profiles. In: Proceedings of the 6th International Conference on Pervasive Technologies Related to Assistive Environments, p. 17. ACM (2013)

37. Peek, S.T., Wouters, E.J., Van Hoof, J., Luijkx, K.G., Boeije, H.R., Vrijhoef, H.J.: Factors influencing acceptance of technology for aging in place: a systematic review. Int. J. Med. Inform. **83**(4), 235–248 (2014)

38. Peters, C., Blohm, I., Leimeister, J.M.: Anatomy of successful business models for complex services: insights from the telemedicine field. J. Manag. Inf. Syst. **32**(3), 75–104 (2015)

39. Reginatto, B.M.B.: Understanding barriers to wider telehealth adoption in the home environment of older people: An exploratory study in the irish context. Int. J. Adv. Life Sci. **4**(3) (2012)

40. Sandanayake, T.C.: Promoting open educational resources-based blended learning. Int. J. Educ. Technol. High. Educ. **16**(1), 1–16 (2019). https://doi.org/10.1186/s41239-019-0133-6

41. Siegel, C., Hochgatterer, A., Dorner, T.E.: Contributions of ambient assisted living for health and quality of life in the elderly and care services-a qualitative analysis from the experts perspective of care service professionals. BMC Geriatrics **14**(1), 112 (2014). https://doi.org/10.1186/1471-2318-14-112

42. Sousa, R.T., Teles, S., Bertel, D., Schmitter, P., Abrantes, D.: Back to the roots: the perspectives of multiple stakeholders about a seamless physical virtual AAL advisory service. In: Proceedings of the 5th International Conference on Information and Communication Technologies for Ageing Well and e-Health - Volume 1: ICT4AWE, pp. 146–155. INSTICC, SciTePress (2019). https://doi.org/10.5220/0007762201460155

43. Teles, S., Kofler, A.C., Schmitter, P., Ruscher, S., Paúl, C., Bertel, D.: ActiveAdvice: a multi-stakeholder perspective to understand functional requirements of an online advice platform for AAL products and services. In: Röcker, C., O'Donoghue, J., Ziefle, M., Maciaszek, L., Molloy, W. (eds.) ICT4AWE 2017. CCIS, vol. 869, pp. 168–190. Springer, Cham (2018). https://doi.org/10.1007/978-3-319-93644-4_9

44. Wild, D., Kydd, A., Szczepura, A.: Implementing digital skills training in care homes: a literature review. Nurs. Older People **28**(4) (2016)

The Results of an Iterative Evaluation Process of an Mhealth Application for Rewarding Healthy Behaviour Among Older Adults

Stephanie Jansen-Kosterink[1,2(✉)], Roos Bulthuis[1,2], Silke ter Stal[1,2],
Lex van Velsen[1,2], Aristodemos Pnevmatikakis[3], Sofoklis Kyriazakos[4],
Andrew Pomazanskyi[5], and Harm op den Akker[1,2]

[1] eHealth Group, Roessingh Research and Development, Enschede, The Netherlands
{s.jansen,r.bulthuis,s.terstal,l.vanvelsen,h.opdenakker}@rrd.nl
[2] Biomedical Signals and Systems Group, University of Twente, Enschede, The Netherlands
[3] Multimodal Signal Analytics, Athens Information Technology, Athens, Greece
apne@ait.gr
[4] Department of Business Development and Technology, Aarhus University, Aarhus, Denmark
sofoklis@btech.au.dk
[5] Nurogames GmbH, Cologne, Germany
andrew.pomazanskyi@nurogames.com

Abstract. It is a challenge to find effective ways for supporting older adults to increase their levels of physical activity and develop habitual physical activity behaviours. Within the GOAL project, an mHealth intervention to motivate older adults to be active was developed, by blending the iterative design and the evaluation activities. The aim of this paper is to present the results of the iterative evaluation process of this mHealth intervention. Evaluation end-points were usability, user experience and potential effect. In total, four cycles of evaluation and redesign of GOAL were conducted in order to create value-adding technology, and demonstrate its impact. Each cycle contained test-weeks, weeks for data analysis, and time for technical modification. In total, 28 participants (students and older adults) interacted with GOAL for a total of 476 days and provided their feedback. During the process, various usability issues were solved to improve GOAL. The users rated the usability of GOAL as acceptable. Older adults were positive about the idea to encourage a healthy lifestyle by using GOAL. During the final evaluation cycle, GOAL encouraged older adults to be more active and motivated them to reach their daily goal.

Keywords: Older adults · eHealth · mHealth · Games · Rewards · Iterative design · Usability testing · Evaluation

1 Introduction

Despite the benefits of being physically active, the overwhelming majority of European older adults do not meet the minimum physical activity levels necessary to remain healthy

© Springer Nature Switzerland AG 2020
M. Ziefle and L. A. Maciaszek (Eds.): ICT4AWE 2019, CCIS 1219, pp. 62–78, 2020.
https://doi.org/10.1007/978-3-030-52677-1_4

[1]. Unfortunately, a sedentary lifestyle is currently predominant in European older adults. Among older adults, inactivity and a sedentary lifestyle are linked to numerous negative health outcomes, comparable to the negative health outcomes of smoking, excessive alcohol intake and obesity [2, 3]. Being physically active has many benefits: it prevents the development of chronic health-related problems, it improves psychological well-being and social outcomes [4], and can slow down muscle loss and prevent a decrease in strength [5–7].

It is a challenge to find effective ways to support older adults to increase their level of physical activity and develop habitual physical activity behaviours. It is known that older adults are less interested in improving their health, but more interested in retaining the state of health they already possess [8]. Next to this, they are more interested in intrinsically enjoyable activities, such as group activities [9], as they emphasise fun and enjoyment of social interaction as a motivation to be physically active. The engaging nature of games can also provide motivating and enjoyable means to comply with exercises and to increase physical activity [10, 11]. Games can be provided to older adults in the old-fashioned way, such as board games, but also as mobile applications for their smartphone or tablet. The latter is facilitated by the rapidly increasing use of such technologies for health-related purposes [12] and gamification (the application of game elements to non-game field) can engage older adults to use, and keep using technology [13, 14].

Within the GOAL project, a new mHealth intervention to motivate older adults to be active was developed. This mobile application rewards healthy behaviour, such as being physically active, training the memory and participating in social activities, with GOAL coins [15]. These coins can be used in mobile games. In doing so, GOAL addresses the adoption of mHealth application that remains limited in the older population [16, 17]. To facilitate improvement of GOAL and its uptake by older adults, an iterative approach was followed [18]. In the GOAL development process, this iterative design (where technology is developed, tested, and then redesigned and improved, using multiple iterations) and evaluation activities blended into each other. The aim of this paper is to present the results of the iterative evaluation of an mHealth application for rewarding healthy behaviour among older adults on usability, user experience and potential effect.

2 Methods

In order for a technology to be pleasurable and meaningful, and thus, to be a success, it must be first and foremost be functional and reliable. In other words, the tool must work from a technological point of view. Then, when it is deemed functional and reliable, one can focus on usability. Only when functionality, reliability, and usability are evaluated to a satisfactory degree, the focus can shift to the user experience (including acceptance). For the evaluation of GOAL, we took a similar approach. When we test the technology with the target group (i.e., older adults), we want to make sure that the technology is of such a quality that it works properly and has a minimum level of usability. In order to achieve the latter, two evaluations were conducted in which participants with a high level of digital literacy interacted with GOAL. Based on these experiences, the usability and user experience of GOAL were improved. We applied this approach, so as not to burden a vulnerable population with low digital literacy (older adults) with a technology that had potential usability flaws, which could easily be identified by conducting tests with an easy to find, non-vulnerable group of participants. Only when we were sure that GOAL functioned properly on a technological level, and had an acceptable level of usability, did we embark on tests with older adults.

2.1 The GOAL Technology

From the point of view of the end-user, GOAL consists of the two core components: the GOAL website and the GOAL mobile application. The Website is the "entry-point" to the platform. This website leads the end-user to a signup page for new users. Within the website the end-user is able to set up an account or log in using already existing credentials. Upon registration or login, the user is exposed to the main dashboard of the web application from which they are able to navigate to the main sections of the application including the wallet (providing an overview of GOAL coin transactions), the physical activity dashboard, games and access to a social marketplace.

The GOAL mobile application is the information centre that the user can use to get all GOAL-related info and access the different GOAL services. It offers users' profile management, an overview of the gained GOAL coins, an overview and access to the games and an overview of the social marketplace tasks. Uniquely for the mobile version, it also offers physical activity tracking. The information is summarized in an overview screen, from where the user can navigate to screens with additional details (see Fig. 1). In an earlier paper the GOAL technology is described in more detail [15].

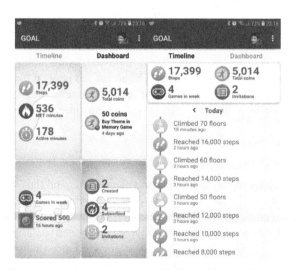

Fig. 1. Overview screen of the GOAL Mobile Application.

2.2 Overview of the Evaluation Cycles

In total, four cycles of evaluation and redesign of GOAL were conducted in order to 1) create value-adding technology, and 2) to demonstrate its impact. Every cycle contained test-weeks and weeks for analysis of test data and technical modification. Table 1 displays the different cycles, their aim, the methods that were applied and the participants that were recruited in each cycle.

Table 1. Overview of the aim, methods and participants of each evaluation cycles.

Cycle	Aim	Method (s)	Participants
1	Usability	Pretest: demographics and think aloud protocol Post-test: exit interview and questionnaires	Students
2	Usability	Pretest: demographics and think aloud protocol Post-test: exit interview and questionnaires	Students
3	Usability and user experience	Pretest: demographics and think aloud protocol Post-test: exit interview and questionnaires	Older adults
4	Usability, user and game experience and potential effect	Pretest: demographics Post-test: exit interview and questionnaires	Older adults

3 Cycle 1

Participants were asked to complete a pre-test assessment. First, they were asked to complete a short demographics questionnaire. Then, a concurrent think-aloud protocol was administered in which they had to complete four predefined tasks within GOAL while verbalizing their thoughts. The data acquired in this way was supplemented by the observations of a researcher. The tasks included:

- Task 1: Downloading the GOAL mobile application.
- Task 2: Setting up an account.
- Task 3: Visiting the GOAL website.
- Task 4: Pairing the GOAL mobile application with the external Activity Coach application.

These tasks reflected some of the central functionalities of GOAL. Participants had five minutes to complete each task. If they could not complete the task within that time or did not want to proceed, they proceeded to the next task. After carrying out all tasks, they filled out the System Usability Scale (SUS) [19].

During this first cycle of the evaluation, participants were asked to use GOAL for 7 days. After these 7 days, participants were invited for a post-test assessment. This post-test assessment started with a short semi-structured interview, in which participants were asked to share their ideas about GOAL. We discussed the advantages, the points of improvement and the experienced problems. After the semi-structured interview, participants were asked to complete the SUS again.

Both the pre- and post-test assessment had an average length of 30 min. The tests were conducted in a usability lab. Each test was performed in a closed room to minimize distraction. Audio recordings were made during the tests. All participant gave informed consent prior to pre- or post-test assessment.

3.1 Technology

During the first cycle, a basic version of GOAL was used. This version included the GOAL mobile application and the Activity Coach application. The GOAL mobile application consisted of a dashboard presenting four functionalities: activity tracking, coin collecting, playing games, and challenging other users. The Activity Coach is a mobile application that can be paired with a commercial activity tracker and digital weighing scale to count steps and track weight. Next to the mobile application, the end-user had access to the GOAL website. This website leads the end-user to a signup page for new users. Within the website, the end-user is able to set up an account or log in using already existing credentials.

3.2 Participants

In total, ten participants were recruited for the first cycle of the GOAL evaluation. In the Netherlands five participants were recruited for pre- and post-test, although one did not participate in the post-test. In Greece, five participants were recruited who only participated in the post-test evaluation. During the evaluation of GOAL, we did not want to unnecessarily burden the target population (community dwelling older adults). As the maturity level was uncertain and multiple usability issues were expected, students and colleagues were asked to participate. Of the all participants, four were male and six were female. Their age was, on average, 29 years (range between 23 and 41 years old).

3.3 Pre-test Assessment

Usability Issues: During the pre-test, the participants had problems with executing the four basic tasks. Participants had problems with finding the GOAL mobile application in the Google Play Store. Additionally, participants preferred receiving feedback when having successfully registered. Participants also indicated that they were unaware of the term "stride length". However, participants thought the ability to update their profile through the settings menu was intuitive. When going to the website, participants noticed that it was not optimized for use on the mobile phone, although they indicated they would like to use the website on their phone. They would find it convenient to have a link to the website in the mobile application.

Usability: Pre-test, the GOAL mobile application SUS scored was between 28 and 75 points. The average score on the SUS was 55 (SD 20.2) indicating that the usability is "ok".

3.4 Post-test Assessment

Praise for the GOAL Platform: The participants liked the potential to get a reward for being active. They indicated that it would be fun to track activities and set goals. The participants also liked the user interface of the mobile application, which, they stated, was easy to use and intuitive. One participant indicated that this mobile application could be possible interesting for children, especially when they are physically inactive.

Usability Issues: The participants indicated that none of the options were functional. The step counter did not work for them, it was unclear if they needed an external activity monitor to count steps, the participants could not collect any coins or set goals/tasks, and the games were not available yet.

Usability: Post-test, the SUS score changed, the four participants recruited in the Netherlands rated the GOAL mobile application between 43 and 68 and an average score of 56 (SD 10.5, n = 4). Together with the five participants from Greece, the usability of the GOAL mobile application was rated "ok" (SUS score 70 (SD 17.6)).

4 Cycle 2

For the second cycle of the GOAL evaluation, we followed the same methods as described for the first cycle. However, one of the tasks to be performed during the pre-test to assess the usability of GOAL was changed (task 4). The participants had to complete the following four tasks:

- Task 1: Downloading the GOAL mobile application.
- Task 2: Setting up an account.
- Task 3: Visiting the GOAL website.
- Task 4: Pairing the GOAL mobile application with one of the available games ("Let's Quiz!" or "Pair me!").

4.1 Technology

During the second cycle, a GOAL mobile application with several updates (mainly bug fixing) was used. This version of the GOAL mobile application could be paired with the Activity Coach and could be paired with two games that could be downloaded from the Google Play store: "Let's Quiz!" and "Pair Me!"

4.2 Participants

Considering the outcome of the first cycle of the GOAL evaluation and the number of requests for improvement, we decided to invite students to participate again. To evaluate the improvements of the GOAL platform, the participants of the first cycle were asked to also participate in this second cycle. Additionally, new participants were recruited in both the Netherlands and Greece. In total, 13 participants completed the second cycle. Of the participants, 5 were male. Their average age was 29.1 years old (range of 16–47 years).

4.3 Pre-test Assessment

Usability Issues: The participants still had several problems with the execution of the four basic tasks. Participants again had problems with finding the GOAL mobile application in the Google Play store, and indicated that it was unclear whether and how they could save the entered profile details. The participants viewed the website on a laptop and found the design nice and clean, with clear headings. Participants liked that they could find the games in the GOAL mobile application, although they would like to receive a confirmation that they successfully connected the game to the GOAL mobile application. It was suggested to integrate the games into one app package with the GOAL mobile application, so no separate downloads would be necessary.

Usability: The GOAL mobile application SUS score was between 40 and 85 points. The average score on the SUS was 61.5 (SD 21.8) indicating that the usability is "ok".

4.4 Post-test Assessment

Praise for the GOAL Platform: The participants who also participated in the first cycle of the GOAL evaluation claimed that the updated mobile application was clearly improved. Setting-up the account was very intuitive, and participants found the explaining texts about stride length and other entries useful. Two games were now available to play and participants enjoyed to play the quiz. Moreover, participants were happy that their scores from the games also appeared in the GOAL mobile application. Participants also liked the way their activity level was represented; the graphs were informative and it was nice to have different representations of activity levels.

Usability Issues: Participants did not collect any coins, nor understood how they could collect coins. Moreover, despite being able to set tasks, it was hard to understand what could be done with them. Some participants mentioned that the step counter did not work at all, others thought it only worked after opening the mobile application, and a few stated that the step counter was not accurate. "Let's Quiz!" appeared to have some bugs; questions were repeated, too hard, or contained errors. Four participants who had already participated in the first cycle, mentioned that they forgot their password and would like a 'password reset' button.

Usability: During the post-test, the SUS scores changed. The nine Dutch participants rate the GOAL mobile application between 32 and 80, with an average score of 58.2 (SD 12.8, n = 9). The four participants from Greece rated the GOAL mobile application between 72.5 and 80, with an average score of 76.3 (SD 3.2, n = 4). Taken together, the post-test SUS score averaged at 65.7 (SD 17.0, n = 13).

5   Cycle 3

For the third cycle of the GOAL evaluation, we followed the same methods as described for the first and second cycle. The tasks to be performed during the pre-test to assess the usability of the GOAL platform were the same. However, to assess the end-user experience we asked the participants to complete post-test after the short semi-structured interview a questionnaire focusing on end-user experience. This questionnaire with summated rating scales was based on the Technology Acceptance Model (TAM) [20]. We expanded TAM with factors that have been found to shape the user experience of mHealth technology: enjoyment [21], aesthetics [22], control [23], and trust in the technology [24].

5.1   Technology

During the third cycle, a GOAL mobile application with several updates was used. The features of the GOAL mobile application were expanded. In this version the activity tracking was optimized by the option to switch for activity tracking to the Activity Coach app (which incorporates steps data from a Fitbit tracker). Next to this, improvements were made to various charts to present GOAL activities and the level of daily activity to the user. Last, in this version of the GOAL mobile application it was feasible to manually create and reward tasks within the social marketplace.

5.2   Participants

After cycle 1 and 2 of the GOAL evaluation, the maturity level of the technology was sufficient to ask community dwelling older adults to use the technology for a longer period of time (1 week). In total, eight participants completed the third cycle. Initially, fifteen community dwelling older adults agreed to participate, but three owned an incompatible smartphone, two did not have or did not use a smartphone, one decided to withdraw, and one had health problems during the evaluation sessions. Two participants were female. The average age was 72 (range 69–76) and five participants completed higher education. The participants were members of a panel that is aimed to involve older adults in eHealth design.

5.3   Pre-test Assessment

Usability Issues: During the pre-test, seven participants managed to download and install the mobile application. One participant did not manage to do so. Some participants mentioned they had never used the Google play store to download and install a mobile application. When creating an account, the participants struggled with finding the registration screen and typing the password twice, and two participants asked whether the password needed to fulfil requirements. The GOAL mobile application crashed several times when attempting to fill in the user's weight in the profile section, and many participants struggled with filling in the profile details (they had trouble with finding the next profile section, saving the profile details, and scrolling to the right date of birth). When going to the GOAL website on a computer, four participants managed to find the login page without help. Logging on to the website appeared to be troublesome, because many participants could not read where to enter the details, due to a low contrast between letters and background. Two participants wanted to have bigger letters, but three older adults indicated they liked the simple design. Two older adults did not understand how to return to the main dashboard. All participants could install the game and login, although the login screen was unintuitive.

Usability: The GOAL mobile application SUS score was between 55 and 80 points. The average score on the SUS was 70 (SD 8.5) indicating that the usability is "ok".

5.4 Post-test Assessment

Praise for the GOAL Platform: Half of the participants enjoyed the games, and three older adults indicated they would like to use the mobile application if it would actually count steps accurately. The dashboard was perceived as simple and basic, with a nice overview of everything. Older adults also enjoyed looking at how many steps they took, with one person considering the idea of collecting coins for fun.

Usability Issues: Five participants indicated that the step counter did not work and did not count steps at all. Two participants indicated that they do not carry their phone all the time, and one would prefer to have a watch. Some participants did not understand MET minutes, the red line in the activity graph, and two participants preferred more explanations about the menu and functions of the GOAL mobile application. Three participants indicated they would like to record cycling as well, and a Dutch mobile application version was also preferred. The participants did not specifically like collecting coins, and many did not collect coins as their step counter did not work. None of them used coins in the games. Two older adults forgot their password and could not use the memory game.

Usability: At the post-test, the SUS score changed. The eight participants rated the GOAL mobile application between 40 and 87.5, with an average score of 65.6 (SD 15.7, $n = 8$). This is slightly lower than pre-test score.

User Experience: The scores on the user experience are presented in Table 2. Indicating the wide range, the opinions of the participants were very diverse. Overall, their opinion on the user experience determinants was neutral. However, five participants indicated that the mobile application was "easy to use".

Table 2. User experience score of evaluation cycle three.

	Range	Average	Attitude of participants (n) towards the GOAL platform		
			Positive	Neutral	Negative
Enjoyment	1.8–4.5	3.3 (SD ± 0.9)	1	7	0
Aesthetics	1.5–5.4	3.4 (SD ± 1.1)	1	6	1
Control	2.0–6.7	4.0 (SD ± 1.6)	2	4	2
Trust in technology	2.0–4.5	3.4 (SD ± 0.8)	1	7	0
Perceive usefulness	2.0–5.0	3.0 (SD ± 1.1)	3	5	0
Ease of use	1.0–6.0	3.0 (SD 2.0)	5	2	1
Intention to use	1.8–4.5	3.3 (SD ± 0.9)	1	7	0

5.5 Focus Groups

During cycle 3 of the GOAL evaluation, we also discussed GOAL with a group of older adults from a local elderly association. After an introduction of the GOAL technology, the older adults were asked to share the advantages and disadvantages they saw, and their ideas concerning the possibility to earn GOAL points.

In total, 21 older adults participated during the two focus groups. The majority of the participants were male (62%). The average age of participants was 72 years old (SD ± 3.7 years; range 64–79 years-old). As advantages, the majority of the participants (52%) mentioned the aim of the technology to encourage a healthy lifestyle. Next to this, seven participants mentioned that the fact that GOAL is free to use (no financial reimbursement). Another five participants mentioned that they liked the idea to learn something new and experienced using GOAL as fun or a nice challenge. As disadvantages, participant mentioned the fact that the GOAL mobile application is only available for Android smartphones (nine participants) and that the GOAL mobile application is mainly in English (five participants). As another disadvantage it was mentioned that the target population is partly reluctant towards playing mobile games (five participants).

Thirteen participants, claimed that maintaining health could be the biggest reward when using GOAL. Another reward that was mentioned is "making progression visible" (by seven participants). Next to this, four participants experienced being active as a reward in and of itself. With respect to earning GOAL coins, eight participants claimed that they wanted to earn GOAL coins by being physically active. Last, the participants were asked how they would like to spend the GOAL points they earned. Nine participants would like to receive a gift card for (digital) books/newspapers (n = 3), for things related to their hobby (n = 5), or to buy new technology (n = 1). Four participants would like to help others or a charity, one participant would like to spend coins on activities with his/her grandchildren, and one participant would like to receive a discount on his/her health insurance. Finally, eight participants had no interest in spending earned GOAL coins.

6   Cycle 4

Various improvements were made after the third cycle. As the primary focus of cycle 3 was on usability and user experience, limited data was gathered on the actual use of the technology. Therefore, cycle 4 focused on the use of GOAL by the target population (community dwelling older adults) with pre-installed technology on a Samsung S3 smartphone and a Fitbit Alta step counter. During pre-test, participants were instructed on how to use the smartphone with the pre-installed mobile application and the Fitbit. They put the Fitbit on their wrist and were told to synchronize the Fitbit with the smartphone every day. During pre-test, the participants completed several questionnaires:

- The revised Sports Motivation Scale (SMS-II) [25], a validated instrument for assessing sports motivation; a domain closely related to adopting a healthy lifestyle. [26]
- The Physical Activity Scale (PAS) [27], a scale in which respondents indicated the hours per day spent in nine different activity categories, ranging from sleeping and resting, to running and playing tennis.
- A health literacy questionnaire [28], with three questions three focused on respondents' confidence and need for help in understanding health information

The participants were asked to use the Fitbit and smartphone for at least two weeks in their normal life. They could use the GOAL mobile application at their own discretion. A post-test assessment was scheduled fourteen days later. During the post-test interview, participants expressed their general experience with the GOAL application, completed the System Usability Scale, and the TAM section of the User Experience Questionnaire from previous cycles, with the addition of several questions on likeability and motivation. Last, during a semi-structured interview, participants addressed the separate components of GOAL. The post-test assessment had an average length of 45 min. Audio recordings were made during the tests. All participants gave informed consent prior to pre-test assessment.

6.1   Technology

During the fourth cycle, a GOAL mobile application with several updates was used. The social marketplace feature was improved extensively. For instance, task invitations could be ignored, task creators could delete pending tasks and past tasks were listed in a new screen. Next to this, there was a redesign of the UI of the GOAL mobile application and bugs were fixed. Last, a gamification layer (Island Exploration game) was available. This game rewarded end-users with mini games when the daily step goal was reached.

6.2   Participants

In total, fifteen participants were included in this evaluation. Seven of them also participated in the third evaluation cycle. Of these participants, eight were male and seven were female. Their average age was 69.6 ± 5.4 years (range 59–78). Nine participants completed higher education, and fourteen lived together with a partner. All participants answered the eleven questions regarding their motivation to live healthy [26]. From this questionnaire, it appeared that eleven participants were intrinsically motivated to live healthy. The average health literacy score was 0.76 ± 0.1 on a 0–1 scale. The average estimated MET (metabolic equivalent) per 24-h day was 46.4 ± 8.2 (range 31.1–58.2), which falls right below the 49.66 as measured by Aadahl and Jørgensen [27] in 39 Danish men and women from the age range 20–60.

6.3 Post-test Assessment

Praise for the GOAL Platform: Most participants enjoyed seeing their step count and activity level and many of them were motivated to go for a walk if they saw that they had a low step count. Even older adults who indicated they were not motivated by the numbers, stated that they sometimes went for an extra walk to make some additional steps. Meeting the step goal was challenging for some, but older adults also enjoyed reaching their goal.

Some participants mentioned they enjoyed playing the games; especially Let's Quiz received positive feedback. Pair Me was also perceived as fun and a few older adults indicated they enjoyed the mini game in the Island Exploration game. One person would definitely buy the GOAL mobile application if it became available.

Usability Issues: The participants did not have to install the GOAL mobile application themselves, so no feedback could be provided on downloading and installing the app. Each participant used the GOAL mobile application in combination with a Fitbit that needed to be synchronized with the smartphone using the Fitbit app every day. This caused some problems, as the Bluetooth connection between the Fitbit and the smartphone did not always work.

Unfortunately, technical problems biased the opinion of some participants, while other participants experienced fewer problems. Using the Fitbit also influenced the feedback, since several participants only checked their step count on the Fitbit watch and app, as they said it was easier.

Some participants had technical problems with receiving GOAL coins in the GOAL mobile application. However, many of them expressed that they did not look at how many coins they collected, so they did not notice that they had not received any. Some other participants, who had not this technical problem, also indicated they did not look at the number of coins they received. Reasons for this were that they did not know what to do with these coins, they received too many coins for it to be interesting, or earning coins did not motivate them to be more active and/or use GOAL.

Usability: The GOAL mobile application scored between 27.5 and 97.5 points on the SUS (n = 15). The average score on the SUS was 68 ± 15 indicating that the usability is "ok".

User Experience: The score on the user experience are presented in Table 3. As can be seen from the wide range, the opinions of the participants (n = 15) were very diverse.

Willingness to Pay: Participants indicated their willingness to pay by choosing from the following options: One time 0, 5 or 10 euros, and 2, 5 or 10 euros per months. Very

Table 3. User experience score of the cycle 4.

	Range	Average	Attitude of participants (n) towards the GOAL platform		
			Positive	Neutral	Negative
Ease of use	1–6.5	3.8 ± 1.8	4	8	3
Intention to use	1–7	3.9 ± 1.7	4	8	3
Perceived usefulness	1.5–6	3.2 ± 1.1	3	11	1

few participants (n = 2) would be interested in paying a monthly fee. Six participants were interested to pay a onetime fee of 5 euro (n = 3) or 10 euro (n = 3) and also six participants were not willing to pay for the GOAL mobile application at all.

Gaming Experience: The opinions about games being included in GOAL were diverse. Some participants indicated that they enjoyed the memory game and almost half of the older adults had played the quiz and thought it was fun to do. The older adults who had played the quiz made the following comments: The questions do not fit the target group, the same questions appear repeatedly after a while, and the font size is too small for comfortable reading. The memory game caused problems, as participants claimed that they were logged out of the game and found it too much trouble to log in again. The Island Exploration game lacked an explanation; participants indicated that they did not know how to start a mini game, or how to play it.

We also asked the participants how they liked the separate components GOAL. They rated the GOAL mobile application, PairMe!, Let's Quiz, and the GOAL Island Exploration game on a scale of 1 to 7 (very fun to very dull). The scores are presented in Table 4.

Table 4. Likeability scores for the four components GOAL.

	Range	Average (1 = very fun, 7 = very dull)
GOAL mobile application	1–6	3.1 ± 1.8
PairMe	1–5	3.2 ± 1.1
Let's quiz	1–6	3.3 ± 1.7
Island exploration game	1–6	3.6 ± 1.4

Motivation: The participants indicated how they were motivated by the GOAL mobile application to be more active and rated three statements on a scale of 1 (completely agree) to 7 (completely disagree) (Table 5). It became apparent that participants feel motivated by GOAL in general, but not by collecting coins or by playing the Island Exploration game.

Table 5. Scores on three statements about motivation to be more active.

	Range	Average (1 = agree, 7 = disagree)
GOAL motivated me to be more active	1–5	2.5 ± 1.6
Receiving GOAL COINS motivated me to be more active	4–7	5.1 ± 1.3
The Island Exploration game motivated me to be more active	4–7	5.1 ± 1.2

7 Discussion

The aim of this paper is to present the outcomes of the iterative development and evaluation of an mHealth application for rewarding healthy behaviour among older adults. In total, 28 participants (students and older adults) interacted with GOAL for 476 days and provided their feedback for improving the technology. During the iterative cycles, various usability issues were solved to improve the usability of the GOAL platform. In the end, the usability of the GOAL platform was acceptable. The aim of GOAL is to motivate the target population (older adults) to live an active life. During the focus groups, the majority of the participants were positive about the idea to encourage a healthy lifestyle by using GOAL. And during the final evaluation cycle, most participants enjoyed seeing their step count and activity level and many were motivated to go for a walk if they saw that they had a low step count. Older adults enjoyed reaching their goal and felt motivated by GOAL in order to be more active.

For this study an iterative approach was followed. In four iterations, the technology was developed, evaluated with end-users, and redesigned. An advantage of this approach is the possibility to tailor GOAL to the specific environment and skills of the older adults. This will, following Broens et al. 2007 [29], maximize the probability of successful implementation. However, successful implementation of technology is not a purely technical topic and multiple aspects need to be taken into account. In general, the acceptance of technology by older adults is based on four aspects: individual aspects, technology aspects, social aspects and delivery aspects [30]. During our evaluations, we mainly focused on technology factors (design and functional features that affect how older adults interact with technology) and individual factors (characteristics of older adults as individual users that affect their interactions with technology). To get a broad overview of the acceptance of GOAL by the older adults it will be good to focus in further studies on the social (expectations and needs that arise from the social and cultural contexts that older adults are in) and delivery (ways in which technology is communicated and distributed to older adults for purchase and use) factors.

An iterative approach is an important component in the development and successful acceptance of eHealth [18]. However, it is not very common in the literature on usability testing to address multiple iterations in one study. A recent scoping review by Maramba et al. 2019 [31] found that in less than a third of the included studies at least two iterations were discussed. This could be due to the possibility that iterations had already taken place prior to the study has being reported [31]. It would be valuable when this kind of information was reported and more information was provided on previous iterations.

As participating in this evaluation of GOAL was voluntary, the selection bias of the subjects is a weakness of this study. The majority of the older adults who were willing to participate, were technology-minded and had the basic skills to use a (smart) phone, tablet or laptop. To assess the usability of GOAL we used the SUS. It was recently found that this instrument is not optimal as a stand-alone usability benchmark for eHealth [32]. Therefore, we also assessed the usability of GOAL by a Think-Aloud protocol to determine the usability issues. For this protocol the participants had to complete several takes, unfortunately we did not report on the task completions or the time to complete the requested task, as this would be a more mature method to test the usability of GOAL.

8 Conclusion

In this paper we have reported on a series of evaluations of different prototypical versions of GOAL. Results show that usability and user experience are satisfactory, but that there is still room for improvement. Results on potential effectiveness suggest that the technology can fulfil its goal: making older adults more active and lead a healthier lifestyle. Combined with the fact that there is willingness to pay shows that the concept of GOAL is evaluated positively, and that, at the current moment, the technology has a satisfactory maturity level.

Acknowledgments. Special thanks go to the subjects who participated in this study, to Mattienne van der Kamp for his assistance in carrying out this study and to the technology developers of RRD, AIT, AU and NG. The GOAL project (H2020 project no. 731656) is an EC-funded project under the call ICT-24-2016: *Gaming and gamification.*

References

1. McPhee, J.S., French, D.P., Jackson, D., Nazroo, J., Pendleton, N., Degens, H.: Physical activity in older age: perspectives for healthy ageing and frailty. Biogerontology **17**(3), 567–580 (2016)
2. Booth, F.W., Gordon, S.E., Carlson, C.J., Hamilton, M.T.: Waging war on modern chronic diseases: primary prevention through exercise biology. J. Appl. Physiol. (Bethesda, Md: 1985) **88**(2), 774–787 (2000)
3. Lee, I.M., Shiroma, E.J., Lobelo, F., Puska, P., Blair, S.N., Katzmarzyk, P.T.: Effect of physical inactivity on major non-communicable diseases worldwide: an analysis of burden of disease and life expectancy. Lancet (London, England) **380**(9838), 219–229 (2012)
4. Bauman, A., Merom, D., Bull, F.C., Buchner, D.M., Singh, M.A.F.: Updating the evidence for physical activity: summative reviews of the epidemiological evidence, prevalence, and interventions to promote "Active Aging". Gerontol. **56**(Suppl 2), S268–S280 (2016)
5. Mijnarends, D.M., et al.: Validity and reliability of tools to measure muscle mass, strength, and physical performance in community-dwelling older people: a systematic review. J. Am. Med. Dir. Assoc. **14**(3), 170–178 (2013)

6. Tak, E., Kuiper, R., Chorus, A., Hopman-Rock, M.: Prevention of onset and progression of basic ADL disability by physical activity in community dwelling older adults: a meta-analysis. Ageing Res. Rev. **12**(1), 329–338 (2013)
7. Zaleski, A.L., et al.: Coming of age: considerations in the prescription of exercise for older adults. Methodist DeBakey Cardiovasc. J. **12**(2), 98–104 (2016)
8. Lockenhoff, C.E., Carstensen, L.L.: Socioemotional selectivity theory, aging, and health: the increasingly delicate balance between regulating emotions and making tough choices. J. Pers. **72**(6), 1395–1424 (2004)
9. Devereux-Fitzgerald, A., Powell, R., Dewhurst, A., French, D.P.: The acceptability of physical activity interventions to older adults: a systematic review and meta-synthesis. Soc. Sci. Med. **2016**(158), 14–23 (1982)
10. Taylor, M.J., McCormick, D., Shawis, T., Impson, R., Griffin, M.: Activity-promoting gaming systems in exercise and rehabilitation. J. Rehabil. Res. Dev. **48**(10), 1171–1186 (2011)
11. Kato, P.M.: Video games in health care: closing the gap. Rev. Gen. Psychol. **14**(2), 113–121 (2010)
12. Gordon, N.P., Hornbrook, M.C.: Older adults' readiness to engage with eHealth patient education and self-care resources: a cross-sectional survey. BMC Health Serv. Res. **18**(1), 220 (2018). https://doi.org/10.1186/s12913-018-2986-0
13. Minge, M., Bürglen, J., Cymek, D.H.: Exploring the potential of gameful interaction design of ICT for the elderly. In: Stephanidis, C. (ed.) HCI 2014. CCIS, vol. 435, pp. 304–309. Springer, Cham (2014). https://doi.org/10.1007/978-3-319-07854-0_54
14. de Vette, F., Tabak, M., Dekker-van Weering, M., Vollenbroek-Hutten, M.: Engaging elderly people in telemedicine through gamification. JMIR Serious Games **3**(2), e9–e9 (2015)
15. Jansen-Kosterink, S., et al.: GOAL: an eHealth application for rewarding healthy behaviour. The first experiences of older adults. In: Proceedings of the 5th International Conference on Information and Communication Technologies for Ageing Well and e-Health, ICT4AWE, vol. 1, ISBN 978-989-758-368-1, pp. 58–66 (2019)
16. Heart, T., Kalderon, E.: Older adults: are they ready to adopt health-related ICT? Int. J. Med. Inform. **82**(11), e209–e231 (2013)
17. Mitzner, T.L., et al.: Technology adoption by older adults: findings from the PRISM trial. Gerontol. **59**(1), 34–44 (2019)
18. van Velsen, L., Evers, M., Bara, C.-D., Op den Akker, H., Boerema, S., Hermens, H.: Understanding the acceptance of an eHealth technology in the early stages of development: an end-user walkthrough approach and two case studies. JMIR Formativ. Res. **2**(1), e10474 (2018)
19. Brooke, J.: SUS - a quick and dirty usability scale. In: Jordan, P.W., Thoma, B., Weerdmeester, B.A. (ed.) Usability Evaluation in Industry, pp. 189–194. Taylor & Francis, London (1995)
20. Davis, F.D.: Perceived usefulness, perceived ease of use, and user acceptance of information technology. MIS Q. **13**(3), 319–340 (1989)
21. Crutzen, R., Cyr, D., de Vries, N.K.: Bringing loyalty to e-Health: theory validation using three internet-delivered interventions. J. Med. Internet Res. **13**(3), e73 (2011)
22. Baumel, A., Muench, F.: Heuristic evaluation of ehealth interventions: establishing standards that relate to the therapeutic process perspective. JMIR Ment. Health **3**(1), e5 (2016)
23. Hawkins, R.P., Han, J.Y., Pingree, S., Shaw, B.R., Baker, T.B., Roberts, L.J.: Interactivity and presence of three eHealth interventions. Comput. Hum. Behav. **26**(5), 1081–1088 (2010)
24. Van Velsen, L., Wildevuur, S., Flierman, I., Van Schooten, B., Tabak, M., Hermens, H.: Trust in telemedicine portals for rehabilitation care: an exploratory focus group study with patients and healthcare professionals. BMC Med. Inform. Decis. Mak. **16**(1), 11 (2016)
25. Pelletier, L.G., Rocchi, M.A., Vallerand, R.J., Deci, E.L., Ryan, R.M.: Validation of the revised sport motivation scale (SMS-II). Psychol. Sport Exerc. **14**(3), 329–341 (2013)

26. van Velsen, L., Broekhuis, M., Jansen-Kosterink, S., op den Akker, H.: Tailoring persuasive eHealth strategies for older adults on the basis of personal motivation: an online survey (preprint). J. Med. Internet Res. **21**, e11759 (2018)
27. Aadahl, M., Jorgensen, T.: Validation of a new self-report instrument for measuring physical activity. Med. Sci. Sports Exerc. **35**(7), 1196–1202 (2003)
28. Chew, L.D., Bradley, K.A., Boyko, E.J.: Brief questions to identify patients with inadequate health literacy. Fam. Med. **36**(8), 588–594 (2004)
29. Broens, T.H., Huis in't Veld, R.M., Vollenbroek-Hutten, M.M., Hermens, H.J., van Halteren, A.T., Nieuwenhuis, L.J.: Determinants of successful telemedicine implementations: a literature study. J. Telemed. Telec. **13**(6), 303–309 (2007)
30. Lee, C., Coughlin, J.F.: PERSPECTIVE: older adults' adoption of technology: an integrated approach to identifying determinants and barriers. J. Prod. Innov. Manag. **32**(5), 747–759 (2014)
31. Maramba, I., Chatterjee, A., Newman, C.: Methods of usability testing in the development of eHealth applications: a scoping review. Int. J. Med. Inform. **126**, 95–104 (2019)
32. Broekhuis, M., van Velsen, L., Hermens, H.: Assessing usability of eHealth technology: a comparison of usability benchmarking instruments. Int. J. Med. Inform. **128**, 24–31 (2019)

Language Complexity in On-line Health Information Retrieval

Marco Alfano[1,5](⊠) ⓘ, Biagio Lenzitti[2] ⓘ, Davide Taibi[3] ⓘ, and Markus Helfert[4] ⓘ

[1] Lero, Dublin City University, Dublin, Ireland
marco.alfano@lero.ie
[2] Dipartimento di Matematica e Informatica, Università di Palermo, Palermo, Italy
biagio.lenzitti@unipa.it
[3] Istituto per le Tecnologie Didattiche, Consiglio Nazionale delle Ricerche, Palermo, Italy
davide.taibi@itd.cnr.it
[4] Lero, Maynooth University, Maynooth, Co. Kildare, Ireland
markus.helfert@lero.ie
[5] Anghelos Centro Studi sulla Comunicazione, Palermo, Italy

Abstract. The number of people searching for on-line health information has been steadily growing over the years so it is crucial to understand their specific requirements in order to help them finding easily and quickly the specific information they are looking for. Although generic search engines are typically used by health information seekers as the starting point for searching information, they have been shown to be limited and unsatisfactory because they make generic searches, often overloading the user with the provided amount of results. Moreover, they are not able to provide specific information to different types of users. At the same time, specific search engines mostly work on medical literature and provide extracts from medical journals that are mainly useful for medical researchers and experts but not for non-experts.

A question then arises: Is it possible to facilitate the search of on-line health/medical information based on specific user requirements? In this paper, after analysing the main characteristics and requirements of on-line health seeking, we provide a first answer to this question by exploiting the Web structured data for the health domain and presenting a system that allows different types of users, i.e., non-medical experts and medical experts, to retrieve Web pages with language complexity levels suitable to their expertise. Furthermore, we apply our methodology to the results of a generic search engine, such as Google, in order to re-rank them and provide different users with the proper health/medical Web pages in terms of language complexity.

Keywords: E-Health · Health information seeking · User requirements · Language complexity · Structured data on the web

1 Introduction

The number of people searching for on-line health information has been steadily growing over the years [1, 2] so it is crucial to understand their specific requirements in order

© Springer Nature Switzerland AG 2020
M. Ziefle and L. A. Maciaszek (Eds.): ICT4AWE 2019, CCIS 1219, pp. 79–100, 2020.
https://doi.org/10.1007/978-3-030-52677-1_5

to help them finding easily and quickly the specific information they are looking for. Although search engines are typically used by health information seekers as the starting point for their searches [2, 3], they have been shown to be limited and unsatisfactory for finding online health information easily and quickly [4, 5]. In particular, generic search engines (e.g., GoogleTM or BingTM) exploit the whole Web but make generic searches, often overloading the user with the offered amount of information. Moreover, they are not able to provide specific information to different types of users. At the same time, specific search engines, such as PubMed[1] or the Cochrane Library[2], mostly work on medical literature and provide extracts from medical journals that are mainly useful for medical researchers and experts but not for non-experts. Moreover, they do not consider all the information contained in the Web that is often addressed to non-medical experts.

A question then arises: Is it possible to facilitate the search of on-line health/medical information based on specific user requirements? In this paper, we provide a first answer to this question by exploiting the structured data on the Web for the health domain and presenting a system that allows different types of users, i.e., non-medical experts and medical experts, to retrieve Web pages with language complexity levels suitable to their expertise. Furthermore, we apply our methodology to a generic search engine, such as Google, in order to re-rank its results and to provide different users with the proper health/medical Web pages in terms of language complexity. To this end, we first present a short survey of the main characteristics and requirements related to health information seeking on the Internet. We then analyze the structured data on the Web with particular reference to the health/medical field (by using *health-lifesci.schema.org*) and classify health Web pages based on different audience types such as patients, clinicians and medical researchers. Next, we present the results of some experiments on the language complexity of medical Web pages with structured data and propose a mapping between the language complexity requirements and the *health-lifesci.schema.org* audience types. We then present the architectural and implementation details of FACILE, a meta search engine that provides Web pages ranked in accordance to the audience type. Finally, we show the results of applying FACILE search and ranking capabilities to both the schema.org structured data and the Google results.

Some of the principles presented in this paper are based on the ones discussed in a previous work [6]. The present work, however, extends the previous study by including a literature survey on the health seekers requirements. Moreover, a larger dataset is used by merging the health-lifesci.schema.org structured data of 2017 with the ones of 2018. Furthermore, the description of the FACILE architecture and implementation (with a new ranking formula that takes into account a higher number of parameters) is added together with the application of the FACILE searching and ranking mechanism to both the *schema.org* structured data and the Google results.

---

[1] https://www.ncbi.nlm.nih.gov/pubmed/

[2] https://www.cochranelibrary.com/

2   Characteristics and Requirements of On-line Health Information Seeking

We now briefly analyze the main characteristics related to health information seeking on the Internet, based on the following dimensions:

- Who (e.g., number of people searching for health information on the Internet);
- Where (e.g., search engines, social networks);
- When (e.g., time frequency);
- What (e.g., symptoms, pathologies, remedies, drugs);
- How (e.g., user requirements of on-line health information seekers).

The 'Cyberchondriacs' Harris Poll [1] shows that the percentage of all US adults who search for health or medical information online has increased from 27% to 76% from 1998 to 2010. Moreover, the 'Health Online 2013' Pew report [2] says that 72% of adult users in the U.S. were looking for health information online in the previous year. When asked to think about the last time they went online for health or medical information, 39% of online health seekers say they looked for information related to their own situation. Another 39% say they looked for information related to someone else's health or medical situation. An additional 15% of these internet users say they were looking both on their own and someone else's behalf. For what concerns Europe, [7] shows a growth from 14% to 39% in the 2005-2007 period. Moreover, in 2010, national bodies reported that 52,5% of adults in Spain were looking for health content on the Internet [8] and 39% in the UK [9].

According to [2], 77% of online health seekers say they began their last session at a search engine such as Google, Bing, or Yahoo. Another 13% say they began at a specialized site in health information, like WebMD. Just 2% say they started their research at a more general site like Wikipedia and an additional 1% say they started at a social network site like Facebook. According to the survey reported in [10], a general search engine is the most frequently used tool to look for online health information. Other popular sources include Websites providing health information (38%) and Wikipedia or medical search tools such as HONselect and Medline Plus (37%). Forums and blogs are always or often used by 23% of the respondents and 5% use Facebook or other social networks. The same paper affirms that Internet is the second source of information after physicians whereas [11] states that Internet is the most commonly consulted resource for health information followed by conversation with health care providers and use of a medical dictionary.

The 'Cyberchondriacs' Harris Poll [1] shows that the percentage of US adults who often or sometimes search for health or medical information online has increased from 42% to 73% from 1998 to 2010. Moreover, 81% of health information seekers say that they have looked for health information online in the last month and 17% say they have gone online to look for health information ten or more times in the last month. On average, health information seekers do this about 6 times a month. According to the survey presented in [10], 24% of the respondents say they look for health information on the Internet at least once a day and 25% do it few times a week. Moreover, 8% do it once a week, 16% do it few times a month and 16% do it once a month.

The 'Health Online 2013' Pew report [2] shows that the most searched health topics are: Specific disease or medical problem (55%), Certain medical treatment or procedure (43%), How to lose weight or how to control your weight (27%), and Health insurance, including private insurance, Medicare or Medicaid (25%). According to the survey reported in [10], the search activity of users is mostly focused on general health information (68%), long-term chronic diseases (59%), healthy lifestyle and nutrition (50%), short-term (up to 2 weeks) acute disease (39%), kids health (22%) and elderly health and care (19%).

A short literature review to evaluate the main user requirements of health information seekers has been carried out in another work [12]. The survey has been revised and extended and the results are reported in Table 1.

Although limited, the literature review presented above shows that the main requirements of health information seekers are the following:

- Language complexity
- Information quality (mainly intended as information trustworthiness)
- Information classification/customization.

Summarizing, we have found that there is a high number of people seeking for health information on the Internet that has been constantly increasing over the years (who). Search engines are the most used means to access medical information (where) and they are used more and more often (when) to seek information on a broad range of medical subjects (what). Moreover, the main requirements of health information seekers are language complexity, information quality and information classification and customization (how).

As stated in the Introduction, this paper mainly focuses on presenting the principles and design/development details of a system that allows to provide different types of users (e.g., medical experts and non-experts) with health/medical Web pages with different language complexity levels so to allow them to immediately find Web medical contents that present a language suitable to their expertise. In another work [12], we explore the other two user requirements, information quality and information classification/customization, and provide a mapping model among those user requirements and the schema.org elements.

As seen in Table 1, the papers dealing with the language complexity user requirement are [10, 13, 16, 17] and [18]. In particular, [10] presents a survey on user requirements which shows that users want to know if the information they search for is explained in the same way their doctor would but they do not present a solution for providing this type of information as we do in this work. Similarly, [13] shows that users feel that the language used must be easy to understand but there is no practical indication on how to achieve it. The system presented in [16] contains a slider that allows to specify the reading level but the system only works with a small amount of information (few pages created by hand) whereas our system automatically works in real time with the health/medical resources provided by *schema.org* (tens of thousands of Web pages) and, in non-real time, with the whole Internet (through Google). [17] suggests that increased understanding can be accomplished by facilitating precise information retrieval with optimized, domain-specific search engines without providing any specific example. They

Table 1. User requirements of health information seekers.

Paper	Language complexity	Info quality	Info classification/customization	Other
N. Pletneva, A. Vargas, C. Boyer. 2011. Requirements for the general public health search [10]	●	●	●	
S. Banna, H. Hasan, P. Dawson. 2016. Understanding the diversity of user requirements for interactive online health services [13]	●	●		
T. Roberts. 2017. Searching the Internet for Health Information: Techniques for Patients to Effectively Search Both Public and Professional Websites [14]		●		
W. Pian, C.S.G. Khoo, J. Chi. 2017. Automatic classification of users' health information need context: Logistic regression analysis of mouse-click and eye-tracker data [15]			●	
P. C.-I. Pang, K. Verspoor, J. Pearce, S. Chang. 2015. Better Health Explorer: Designing for Health Information Seekers [16]	●		●	●
A. Keselman, R. Logan, C. Smith. 2008. Developing informatics tools and strategies for consumer-centered health communication [17]	●	●	●	
S. C. Ardito. 2013. Seeking Consumer Health Information on the Internet [18]	●	●		

also suggest automatic text translation to simpler text in order to enhance text readability. In other works [19, 20], we have also tackled the problem of translating medical/technical terms in lay terms so to facilitate their comprehension by non-medical experts. In the work presented here, however, our system directly finds the easy-to-understand Web pages available on the Web. Finally, [18] lists some consumer medical information reputable sites and suggests that patients should be taught to search PubMed, that is a collection of scientific medical articles mainly devoted to medical researchers. Our system, as already said, exploits the whole Internet and automatically provides either more complex or simpler web content depending on the user requirements.

3 Structured Data in Health Science Domain on the Web

In the last few years the use of *schema.org* vocabularies, to include semantic information in Web pages, has rapidly increased. The *schema.org*[3] initiative has been promoted in 2014 by major players in the search engine market with the aim to create, maintain, and reuse vocabularies for structured data on the Internet. In particular, *schema.org* defines types (e.g., *Product, Organization, People*) and related properties (e.g. *name, title, description*) that are interleaved within the HTML code and used to visualize that information in specific parts of a Web page. At present, the vocabularies defined by *schmea.org* are used in over ten million Web sites and search engines leverage the structured data to provide users with more appropriate results. Along with the core schema, that is used to describe a huge number of different types of entities from learning resources [21, 22] or products and organizations, *schema.org* also defines extensions with the focus on specific sectors such as automotive, Internet of Thing (IoT) and health.

In our study, we are interested in exploiting structured data to match the requirements identified in Sect. 2 with particular respect to the requirements related to the complexity of the language used by the Web pages containing health related information. To this aim, we refer to the *health-lifesci* extension[4] of *schema.org* that contains 93 types, 175 properties and 125 enumeration values related to the health/medical field. They can be used, among others, to extract data related to the requirements of information quality, information classification and language complexity. In particular, for the language complexity, the *MedicalAudience*[5] type plays a key role to identify searching mechanisms that provide targeted information. This type describes the target audiences for medical Web pages and it includes *Patient*[6], *Clinician*[7] and *MedicalResearcher*[8] as more specific types. As reported in *schema.org*, a patient is any person recipient of health care services. Clinicians are medical clinicians, including practicing physicians and other medical professionals involved in clinical practice. Medical researchers are professionals who make research on the medical field.

In order to explore the use of the *schema.org* vocabulary to support health information seeking on the Web, we have evaluated the adoption of the types and properties defined in this vocabulary through the analysis of the *schema.org* information made available by the Web Data Commons initiative. The Web Data Commons (WDC) [23] contains all Microformat, Microdata and RDFa data extracted from the open repository of Web crawl data named Common Crawl (CC). At the time of writing, the latest release of the

---

[3] https://schema.org/.

[4] https://health-lifesci.schema.org/.

[5] http://schema.org/MedicalAudience.

[6] http://schema.org/Patient.

[7] http://schema.org/Clinician.

[8] http://schema.org/MedicalResearcher.

WDC dataset is dated November 2018 and it is based on 2.5 billion crawled pages with about 37% of them including structured data. We extended the work presented in [6] by merging the dataset extracted by WDC in 2017 with the one of 2018. The dataset dumps of the two years are made available by WDC as compressed files (8,433 files for 2017 and 7,263 for 2018). Each file is around 100 MB large and contains information in the form of RDF quadruples. A quadruple is a sequences of RDF terms in the form {s, p, o, u}, where s, p and o represent a triple consisting of subject, predicate, object and u represents the URI of the document from which the triple has been extracted.

Figure 1 presents an example of RDF quads, for the *Patient* subtype, extracted from WDC. It clearly shows the subject, predicate, object and URI of the quadruples. In compliance with the Open Science model, we have made the RDF quads subsets, for the *Patient*, *Clinician* and *MedicalResearcher* specific types, available at the address http://h-easy.lero.ie/opendata/, in order to allow other researchers to use and lead further research on these data.

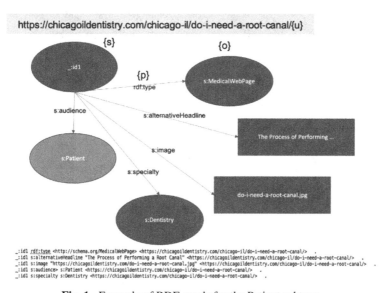

Fig. 1. Example of RDF quads for the Patient subtype.

From the dataset dumps by WDC, we have filtered the quadruples that contain types and properties related to the health domain. The resulting dataset that we have used in our study consists of 103 billion RDF quadruples.

Figure 2 (a) and (b) respectively show the top ten types and properties of the dataset we use for this study. Notice that, although, we have extracted types, properties and enumeration values of health-lifesci.schema.org, some types, such as *Action*, are generic and belong to the *schema.org* core vocabulary, but they assume a specific meaning in the context of *health-lifesci*. For example, the *Action* type is linked to the potential actions of a specific group of drugs. The same applies to properties such as *manufacturer* (presenting the highest frequency) which is generic and belongs to the *schema.org* core vocabulary but, in the context of *health-lifesci,* it refers to the organization producing a specific *Drug.* Finally, notice that Physician is not used as a synonym of doctor but indicates the doctor office[9].

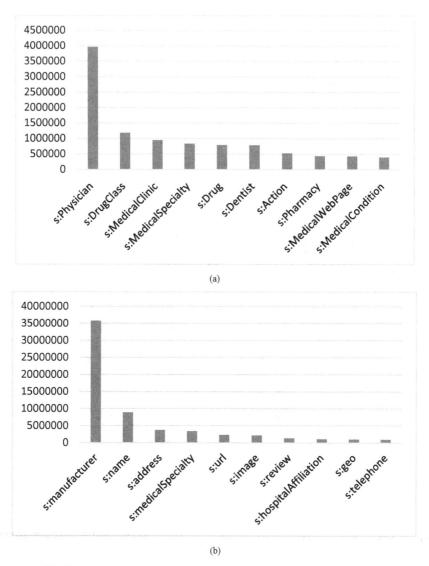

(a)

(b)

Fig. 2. Top ten types (a) and properties (b) of health-lifesci.schema.org.

We have also analyzed the distribution of the so called Pay Level Domains (PLDs) in the dataset including 2017 and 2018 dumps. The complete results of this analysis are

---

[9] https://schema.org/Physician.

available at the address http://h-easy.lero.ie/opendata/ while Table 2 shows the top ten results. In this list, we also indicate whether each PLD is related to the health/medical domain.

Table 2. PLDs with # of quads and health/medical indication.

#quads	PLD	Health/medical
10544968	lybrate.com	Yes
7082432	patents.google.com	No
3346339	vidal.fr	Yes
2556287	vitals.com	Yes
1567948	estdoc.jp	Yes
1368641	restonhospital.com	Yes
1309007	md.com	Yes
1157954	carroya.com	No
1065347	spreadshirt.com	No
957936	doctoranytime.gr	Yes

With regards to the *medicalAudience* property, we have computed the number of quads for each audience types and the results are reported in Table 3.

Table 3. Number of RDF Quads extracted for each specific type.

Schema.org types	RDF quads
Patient	62,251
Clinician	17,416
MedicalResearcher	3,770

These three types, related to *MedicalAudience*, facilitate the identification of pages targeted to patients, clinicians and medical researchers. Table 4 shows an extract of five quads from each subset (the audience appears in the third column).

Notice that, at this stage, we have found Web pages that have been targeted to the different user types by their author, but we do not exactly know the reason behind the choice of considering a page more suitable for a specific audience type. In fact, the motivation could be related to the language complexity level (e.g., more or less technical) or to the treated subject (e.g., pathology symptoms and remedies, for patients, or technical aspects, for medical researchers), or to something else. In the next section, we present a mapping between the language complexity levels and the different audience types so to provide users with Web pages related to their specific requirements.

Table 4. An extract of five RDF quads extracted from Patient (a), Clinican (b) and MedicalResearcher (c) subsets.

Subject	Predicate	Object	Uri
_:genid2d65f95a781e614808bccf de1f41b001c32db0	<http://schema.org/audience>	http://schema.org/Patient	<https://dentistinsurrey.ca/cosm etic-dental-procedures-to-enhance-your-smile/>
<https://medlineplus.gov/spanish/ ency/article/001054.htm>	<http://schema.org/Medic alWebPage/audience>	http://schema.org/Patient	<https://medlineplus.gov/spanis h/ency/article/00105.html>
<https://medlineplus.gov/ency/arti cle/001525.htm>	<http://schema.org/Medic alWebPage/audience>	http://schema.org/Patient	<https://medlineplus.gov/ency/a rticle/001525.htm>
<https://medlineplus.gov/ency/pat ientinstructions/000391.htm>	<http://schema.org/Medic alWebPage/audience>	http://schema.org/Patient	<https://medlineplus.gov/ency/p atientinstructions/000391.htm>
_:node266bc63ad0aaf66daea4a87 983675233	<http://schema.org/Medic alWebPage/audience>	https://health-lifesci. schema.org/Patient	<http://mis-varices-info.es/es/conexiones>

(a)

Subject	Predicate	Object	Uri
_:genid2dde430d3d6a664e879 6b9654a5fa312882db88	<http://schema.org/Medical WebPage/audience>	http://schema.org/Clinician	<https://fpnotebook.com/cv/Ex am/PlsPrdxs.htm>
_:node3651c910a570c21033d 04278bfa589a8	<http://schema.org/Medical WebPage/audience>	http://schema.org/Clinician	<https://fpnotebook.com/cv/Ex am/JPnt.htm>
_:nodebd34e3af7dbf1d2c29d5 20cd3372c32e	<http://schema.org/Medical WebPage/audience>	http://schema.org/Clinician	<https://fpnotebook.com>
_:node76312b2a953eb616b45 ab7fe34f88c	<http://schema.org/Medical ScholarlyArticle/audience>	http://schema.org/Clinician	<http://www.creteilophtalmo.f r/en/2012/neovascularisation-choroidienne-compliquant-une-dmla-atrophique/>
_:node12c5ae94a53b3b39 196fac4bc1aaaa9	<http://schema.org/Medical WebPage/audience>	http://schema.org/Clinician	<http://www.choosingwisely.o rg.au/recommendations/gesa>

(b)

(*continued*)

Table 4. (*continued*)

Subject	Predicate	Object	Uri
_:node4edd6b853592234609 e785dd74bfa28	<http://schema.org/MedicalW ebPage/audience>	http://schema.org/http://sche ma.org/MedicalResearcher	<https://www.malacards.org/>
_:nodea78f8069a42267ba12 6819c0543d237	<http://schema.org/MedicalW ebPage/audience>	http://schema.org/http://sche ma.org/MedicalResearcher	<https://www.malacards.org/c ard/chronic_leukemia>
_:nodeb246e0cf395edb3ff35 64dbf73d916	<http://schema.org/MedicalW ebPage/audience>	http://schema.org/http://sche ma.org/MedicalResearcher	<https://www.malacards.org/se arch/results/atorvastatin>
_:genid2d8ba0b032efee4268 945f68fa2bd1f2442db0	<http://schema.org/audience>	http://schema.org/http://sche ma.org/MedicalResearcher	<https://www.nanostring.com/ products/gene-expression- panels/gene-expression-panels- overview>
_:node57b22f2149e6112a71 febf24e34f9d67	<http://schema.org/MedicalW ebPage/audience>	http://schema.org/http://sche ma.org/MedicalResearcher	https://www.malacards.org/car d/inflammatory_breast_carcino ma

(c)

4   Mapping Language Complexity User Requirements to Audience Types

As seen above, users have different requirements when searching for health information on the Web. In particular, one of the most important requirement for non-expert health information seekers is that the language used in the Web pages must be easy to understand. On the opposite, medical experts require that the info they are looking for presents a proper technical and rigorous terminology. We then consider two classes of users:

- Non experts (e.g., patients or citizens);
- Experts (e.g., physicians or medical researchers).

We have taken the three subsets presented in the previous section, related to *Patient*, *Clinician*, and *MedicalResearcher* audience types, and, for each quadruple, we have analysed the related Web page in order to estimate its language complexity. To this end, we have evaluated the 'term familiarity index', as described in [6, 24, 25] of the English and non-empty Web pages (around 50% of the total). In particular, for each Web page, we have computed the term familiarity of each word by using the number of results provided by the Google search engine and we have then computed the page familiarity index by averaging all the term familiarity indexes. This information has been stored in a database to avoid work duplication.

In particular, for each Web page, we have computed and stored the number of unique words, the related page familiarity, the total number of words and the related page familiarity. The results of the performed experiments, for the three audience types, are available at the address http://www.math.unipa.it/simplehealth/simple2/ResSchema.php and the first six results of each audience type are shown in Fig. 3.

Next, we have computed some statistics related the term familiarity indexes of the Web pages for the different target audiences and we have obtained the results reported in

ID	URL	# Distinct Words	Page Familiarity DW (billions)	# Total Words	Page Familiarity TW (billions)
1	https://tatefamilydentistry.com/...	256	5.95	502	8.51
2	https://midtownoms.com/corrective-jaw-surgery/...	208	5.98	446	8.30
5	https://midtownoms.com/implant-bone-grafting/...	239	4.90	525	8.15
8	https://midtownoms.com/contact-us/...	76	7.80	139	7.18
9	https://www.restylaneusa.com/specialist...	361	4.72	1037	8.60
11	https://midtownoms.com/referring-doctors/...	92	7.56	168	7.68

(a)

ID	URL	# Distinct Words	Page Familiarity DW (billions)	# Total Words	Page Familiarity TW (billions)
3	https://www.onlinedentalmarketing.com/targeted-dental-market...	230	7.03	471	10.35
4	https://www.onlinedentalmarketing.com/targeted-dental-market...	346	5.57	790	9.96
10	https://www.onlinedentalmarketing.com/privacy-policy/...	552	5.36	1422	10.07
16	https://www.onlinedentalmarketing.com/blog/...	299	6.74	664	9.31
18	https://www.onlinedentalmarketing.com/meet-us/...	183	6.59	312	8.28
20	https://www.onlinedentalmarketing.com/targeted-dental-market...	334	5.69	692	9.23

(b)

ID	URL	# Distinct Words	Page Familiarity DW (billions)	# Total Words	Page Familiarity TW (billions)
6	http://hcvhub.deusto.es/	122	6.71	194	8.57
7	http://www.malacards.org/card/geniculate_herpes_zoster...	677	2.39	2047	3.13
15	http://www.malacards.org/card/yaws...	2815	0.87	6994	1.82
37	http://www.malacards.org/card/klippel_feil_syndrome_3_autoso...	314	3.08	1095	2.83
39	http://www.malacards.org/card/chorioretinitis...	2374	0.85	5592	1.67
54	http://www.malacards.org/card/spindle_cell_hemangioma...	555	2.51	1597	3.29

(c)

Fig. 3. First six test results for Patient (a), Clinican (b), and MedicalResearcher (c) audience types.

Fig. 4. It shows, for each specific type, the box plot of the average of the term familiarity indexes computed for all words (page familiarity). A box plot is a standardized way of displaying the distribution of data based on a five-number summary ("minimum", first quartile (Q1), median, third quartile (Q3), and "maximum"). Overall, the median and the first-third quartile interval of *Patient* is much higher of those of *Clinician* and *MedicalResearcher* that partially overlap. The outliers above the maximum mainly refer to pages that contain informative/commercial data for the different types of users and then use a simple language. The outliers below the "minimum" mainly refer to pages, such as those of the www.malacards.org domain, which indicate all three classes, as target audiences, but have a low term familiarity index clearly indicating that they should be targeted only to medical experts for what concerns the language complexity.

The experimental results show that the Web pages targeted to *Patient*, present, on average, a much higher term familiarity index and thus a simpler terminology whereas the Web pages targeted to *Clinician* and *MedicalResearcher* present, on average, a lower term familiarity index and thus a more complex terminology, even though *Clinician* pages are a little closer to *Patient* pages. As a consequence, *Patient* pages, falling in the intervals shown in Fig. 4, can be used for the Non-expert class and *Clinician/MedicalResearcher* pages, falling in the intervals shown in Fig. 4, can be used for the Expert classes producing then the following mapping:

- Non-experts - > *Patient*
- Experts - > *Clinician* and *MedicalResearcher*

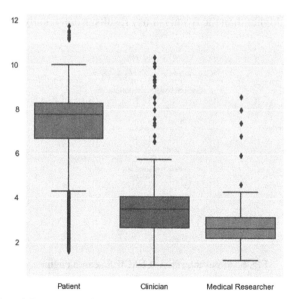

Fig. 4. Box plot of the average of term familiarity indexes for all words (computed in [6]).

This allows us to provide different types of users with health Web pages targeted to their specific language complexity requirements. Notice that the presence of structured data inside a Web page can also be seen, somehow, as a basic guarantee of information quality even though an evaluation of the quality level of a Web page content requires a specific analysis that is outside the scope of this work.

5   FACILE Architecture and Implementation

Once created the mapping model, as shown in the previous Section, we have built a meta search engine, FACILE, that provides the different audience types with the proper Web contents in terms of language complexity. The meta search engine can be accessed at the address http://www.math.unipa.it/simplehealth/facile and Fig. 5 reports the input interface of the engine. Notice that it provides the user with two search possibilities:

- A **Search on Semantic Web (schema.org)** that allows a real-time search by using the health-lifesci.schema.org URLs analysed in the previous sections and allows to specify the audience type, i.e., non-expert (Patient) or expert (Clinician or Medical Researcher);
- A **Search on Google** that uses the Google search engine in order to explore the whole Internet and find the Web pages related to the searched keyword(s) and recomputes the page ranking on the basis of the term familiarity of each Web page. Since this computation takes some time, the search, in this case, is not in real time in the sense that it is not providing the user with an answer in a time comparable to that of a generic search engine. Notice that the interface allows to specify the number of Google results (maximum fifty, higher than the twenty-thirty results usually analysed by a user [26]).

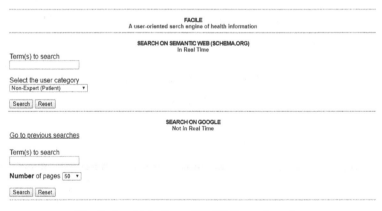

Fig. 5. Input interface of FACILE search engine.

Figure 6 presents the Facile architecture. From top to bottom, we have the following:

- The **Client** allows to search for the medical keyword(s).
- The **Search Engine** behaves slightly differently depending of the two types of search:

  - In the case of **Search on semantic Web (schema.org),** it looks for the lifesci.schema.org URLs related to the keyword(s) into the **FACILE DB** and selects the ones related to the chosen medical audience, i.e., *Patient, Clinician* or *MedicalResearcher*. Moreover, it provides a list of URLs sorted in terms of keyword(s) occurrences and term familiarity (see Sect. 5.1);
  - In the case of **Search on Google**, it first uses Google to find a number of URLs (max 50) related to the keyword. It then uses the **Web page retriever** and **Feature extractor** and loads the results into the **FACILE DB** (this operation requires some time). Finally, it provides a list of URLs sorted in terms of term familiarity (see Sect. 5.2).

- The **FACILE DB**, contains the the information related to the URLs. In the case of the **Search on semantic Web (schema.org)**, each URL is associated to the page words and number of occurrences, the associated medical audience and the page familiarity. In the case of the **Search on Google**, each URL is only associated to the page familiarity.
- The **Web Page Retriever** retrieves Web pages from the Web and the **Feature extractor** extracts/computes page features such number of words, term familiarity, etc.
- The **Health-life.sci.schema.org Quads** contains the quadruples related to *Patient, Clinician*, and *MedicalResearcher* health-lifesci.schema.org elements.

5.1   Use of FACILE with Health-lifesci.chema.org Structured Data

This option, as seen above, gives the user the possibility to input one or more keywords and to indicate the audience, i.e., Non-expert or Expert. The system looks for the lifesci.schema.org URLs related to the keyword(s) into the **FACILE DB** and selects the ones related to the chosen audience. It then provides a list of URLs sorted by using the following ranking formulas:

- Non-Expert (Patient)

$$R = \alpha * (Term\_Occurrences/Max\_Occurrences) + (1-\alpha) \\ *(Page\_Familiarity\_Index)/Max\_Familiarity\_Index) \tag{1}$$

- Expert (Clinician and MedicalResearcher)

$$R = \alpha * (Term\_Occurrences/Max\_Occurrences) - (1-\alpha)* \\ (Page\_Familiarity\_Index)/Max\_Familiarity\_Index) \tag{2}$$

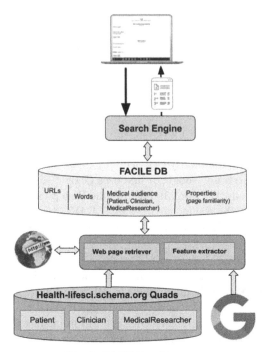

Fig. 6. FACILE architecture.

Where:

- *Term_Occurrences* is the number of occurrences of the keyword(s) in the page;
- *Max_Occurrences* is the maximum number of occurrences of the keyword(s) in all found Web pages;
- *Page_Famililarity_Index* is the page familiarity, i.e., the mean of the term familiarity indexes of the Web page;
- *Max_Famililarity_Index* is the maximum page familiarity of all found Web pages.
- α allows us to differently weighs the number of occurrences and page familiarity.

Notice the non-expert formula is a sum because we want meaningful pages (with high number of occurrences of the searched item) but with the simplest language, whereas the expert formula is a difference because we want meaningful pages (with high number of occurrences of the searched item) but with the most complex/technical language.

We have made some preliminary experiments with the weight and found out that a value of $\alpha = 0.3$ provided us with the best results in terms of correspondence between the intended audience and the provided Web pages. For example, Fig. 7 reports the top ten results of FACILE for the 'diabetes' keyword for the Non-Expert *(Patient)* and Expert *(Clinician and MedicalReseracher)*. For each URL, the number of occurrences of the keyword (diabetes in this case), the page familiarity and the R result of the ranking formula are shown.

By examining Fig. 7 we can easily see that the top links of *Patient* present a high term familiarity index and belong to medlineplus.gov which is notoriously a Web portal for non-experts. The top links of *Clinician* present a medium-low term familiarity index and belong to the fpnotebook.com Web portal - which acts as a medical dictionary - and presents a technical language even though understandable by users with some medical skills or to malacards.org Web portal that is a human disease database and presents a very technical and complex language. The top links of *MedicalResearcher* present a low term familiarity index and belong to malacards.org Web portal that, as said, presents a very technical and complex language. Notice that some malacards.org pages contain all the three audience types and may appear in more than one ranking (as in the case of the *Clinician* and *MedicalResearcher* web pages) because often present a high number of occurrences of the searched item. Of course, the ranking mechanism presented here is just a first proposal and needs to be refined and enriched to transform FACILE in a proper user-oriented search engine. To this end, each result page contains a link to a "detailed page" that presents, among others, the possibility for the user to choose different values of α and thus to experiments with the different ranking possibilities.

5.2   Use of FACILE with Google

The use of structured data related to the intended audience, in combination with the term familiarity of a Web page, provides a method for ranking Web pages in terms of the complexity level of the text. Generalising this approach, the term familiarity analysis can be used for ranking Web pages even when they do not contain any specific structured data about their audience. The **Search on Google** section of the FACILE meta search engine follows this approach by re-ranking the results, obtained through the generic Google search engine, in terms of page familiarity.

An example of this approach is shown in Fig. 8. The results for the "Antibiotics" search keyword in Google, are ranked according to the page familiarity, as provided by FACILE. The table reports each URL with the Google rank and the page familiarity. URLs are ranked by taking into account the page familiarity value of the corresponding Web page, from the highest to the lowest.

The results present a background colour that gives an indication of the intended audience. In particular, the green colour is used to highlight URLs that have a value of page familiarity above 6 that, as seen in Fig. 4, somehow indicates pages suitable to Non-Expert audience. The yellow color is used to indicate URLs that have a value of page familiarity between 5 and 6 and is related to an interval that lies between the Expert or Non-Expert "zone". The red color is used to indicate URLs that have a value of page familiarity below 5, indicating Web pages more suitable, in principle, to an Expert audience.

In our example, the top result is a web page that explains, in lay terms, what antibiotics are and how they work. The other top results of the list refer to nhs.uk and medicalnewsto-day.com domains and also represent Web pages with information for non-expert users. On the opposite, the Web pages appearing at the bottom of the list are related to concepts such as *Tetracycline* and the *Timeline of antibiotics* that use a language more suitable for experts. It is interesting to note how ranking the results according to the term familiarity notably changes the order of the resulting URLs.

1100 PAGES FOR TERM DIABETES OF TYPE PATIENT

Back to Facile Home Page

Details page

#	URL	Occurrences	Familiarity	R.
1	https://medlineplus.gov/ency/article/000305.htm	88	8.54	1.17
2	https://medlineplus.gov/ency/article/000313.htm	86	8.49	1.16
3	https://medlineplus.gov/ency/article/001214.htm	73	8.14	1.08
4	https://medlineplus.gov/ency/patientinstructions/000328.htm	40	9.25	1.07
5	https://medlineplus.gov/ency/patientinstructions/000086.htm	38	9.07	1.04
6	https://medlineplus.gov/ency/patientinstructions/000083.htm	28	8.87	0.99
7	https://medlineplus.gov/ency/patientinstructions/000322.htm	21	9.12	0.99
8	https://medlineplus.gov/ency/patientinstructions/000014.htm	4	9.74	0.99
9	https://medlineplus.gov/ency/patientinstructions/000079.htm	32	8.69	0.98
10	https://medlineplus.gov/ency/article/003640.htm	17	9.10	0.97

(a)

1148 PAGES FOR TERM DIABETES OF TYPE CLINICIAN

Back to Facile Home Page

Details page

#	URL	Occurrences	Familiarity	R
1	http://www.fpnotebook.com/Endo/DM/DbtsMlts.htm	181	3.10	0.29
2	http://www.malacards.org/card/diabetes_mellitus_permanent_neonatal	164	2.56	0.29
3	http://www.malacards.org/card/neonatal_diabetes_mellitus	128	2.09	0.22
4	http://www.malacards.org/card/monogenic_diabetes	143	2.65	0.21
5	http://www.malacards.org/card/diabetes_insipidus_neurohypophyseal	139	2.52	0.21
6	http://www.fpnotebook.com/Endo/DM/DbtcKtcds.htm	118	2.98	0.09
7	http://www.malacards.org/home/malalist/D	41	1.20	0.02
8	http://www.fpnotebook.com/Endo/DM/HyprsmlrHyprglycmcSt.htm	96	3.12	0.01
9	http://www.fpnotebook.com/Renal/Endo/CntrlDbtsInspds.htm	89	3.29	-0.03
10	http://www.malacards.org/card/microvascular_complications_of_diabetes_1	61	2.48	-0.05

(b)

515 PAGES FOR TERM DIABETES OF TYPE MEDICALRESEARCHER

Back to Facile Home Page

Details page

#	URL	Occurrences	Familiarity	R
1	http://www.malacards.org/card/diabetes_mellitus_permanent_neonatal	164	2.56	0.34
2	http://www.malacards.org/card/neonatal_diabetes_mellitus	128	2.09	0.26
3	http://www.malacards.org/card/monogenic_diabetes	143	2.65	0.26
4	http://www.malacards.org/card/diabetes_insipidus_neurohypophyseal	139	2.52	0.26
5	http://www.malacards.org/home/malalist/D	41	1.20	0.03
6	http://www.malacards.org/card/microvascular_complications_of_diabetes_1	61	2.48	-0.02
7	http://www.malacards.org/card/diabetic_polyneuropathy	43	2.18	-0.06
8	http://www.malacards.org/search/results/sepsis?retired=1	6	0.91	-0.07
9	http://www.malacards.org/search/results/ADP	7	0.96	-0.07
10	http://www.malacards.org/search/results/nephritis?retired=1	8	1.03	-0.07

(c)

Fig. 7. Diabetes outputs for *Patient* (a), *Clinician* (b), and *MedicalResearcher* (c).

15 PAGES FOR TERM ANTIBIOTICS

#	URL	Googe Ranking	Familiarity
1	https://microbiologysociety.org/members-outreach-resources/outreach-resources/antibiotics-unearthed/antibiotics-and-antibiotic-resistance/what-are-antibiotics-and-how-do-they-work.html	14	8.55
2	https://www.medicalnewstoday.com/articles/10278.php	1	8.36
3	https://www.nhs.uk/conditions/antibiotics/	12	8.30
4	https://www.drugs.com/article/antibiotics-and-viruses.html	10	8.06
5	https://www.emedicinehealth.com/antibiotics/article_em.htm	15	7.85
6	https://medlineplus.gov/antibiotics.html	11	7.85
7	https://www.nhsinform.scot/tests-and-treatments/medicines-and-medical-aids/types-of-medicine/antibiotics	13	7.77
8	https://www.drugs.com/article/antibiotics-for-uti.html	8	7.35
9	https://www.drugs.com/drug-class/glycopeptide-antibiotics.html	9	6.87
10	https://www.drugs.com/article/antibiotics.html	7	6.74
11	https://en.wikipedia.org/wiki/Antimicrobial	6	6.19
12	https://en.wikipedia.org/wiki/Tetracycline_antibiotics	5	5.61
13	https://en.wikipedia.org/wiki/Antibiotic	2	5.32
14	https://en.wikipedia.org/wiki/Timeline_of_antibiotics	4	4.51
15	https://en.wikipedia.org/wiki/List_of_antibiotics	3	4.11

Fig. 8. Re-ranking Google search for the keyword "Antibiotics".

6 Conclusions

The World Wide Web has more and more become the privileged source for an increasingly number of people looking for health information. The typologies of available information are able to satisfy the needs of different types of users, with different levels of expertise. The wide range of information, from practical suggestions to scholarly papers, matches the requirements of both experts and not experts when it comes to using the Web for health information seeking. However, generic and specialized search engines are not able to immediately and easily provide information to different audience types while, at the same time, exploiting all the health/medical information contained in the Web.

In this work, we have identified the main requirements related to health information seekers on the Web and have proposed an approach to classify Web pages in the health domain that satisfies the language complexity requirement. The proposed approach is based on structured data on the Web. In particular, the *schema.org* vocabulary and, more specifically, the types and properties of its *health-lifesci* extension have been used to classify health Web pages according to the different audience types.

The use of structured data in combination with the evaluation of the term familiarity index has led to a mapping between the language complexity user requirement and the different audience types. Preliminary experiments have been conducted to validate this approach and creating a mapping model. The results of those experiments have guided the design of a meta search engine that allows different users to find Web pages related to their language complexity requirements.

The performed texts and experiments have provided us with satisfying results but a more comprehensive set of tests needs to be undertaken for a evaluating more effectively the correlation between language complexity levels and the different audience types, thus, better identifying the thresholds for what concerns the term familiarity index of a Web page that led to classify the Web page as suitable for experts or non-experts. Moreover, the ranking mechanism of the meta search engine presented here should be refined in order to weight the term familiarity index in combination with the number of the keyword(s) occurrences and other parameters related to further user requirements. The time for re-ranking the Google results also needs to be optimized so to to provide users with results in real or near-real time.

Finally, other user requirements, such as the quality of information and the information classification/customization, have to be taken into account and other types and properties of the schema.org vocabulary have to be included in the proposed method in order to provide users with on-line resources that satisfy the different user requirements and allow them to easily acquire, comprehend and learn health/medical information by exploiting the Web [26–28].

Acknowledgements. This work was partially supported by the European Union's Horizon 2020 research and innovation programme under the Marie Skłodowska-Curie grant agreement No 754489 and by Science Foundation Ireland grant 13/RC/2094 with a co-fund of the European Regional Development Fund through the Southern & Eastern Regional Operational Programme to Lero - the Irish Software Research Centre (www.lero.ie).

References

1. Taylor, H.: HI-Harris-Poll-Cyberchondrics. Harris Interactive (2010). https://theharrispoll.com/the-latest-harris-poll-measuring-how-many-people-use-the-internet-to-look-for-information-about-health-topics-finds-that-the-numbers-continue-to-increase-the-harris-poll-first-used-the-word-cyberch/
2. Fox, S., Duggan, M.: Health Online 2013, Pew, Research Center's Internet & American Life Project (2013). http://www.pewinternet.org/2013/01/15/health-online-2013/
3. Spink, A., et al.: A study of medical and health queries to Web search engines. Health Inf. Libr. J. **21**, 44–51 (2004)
4. Keselman, A., Browne, A.C., Kaufman, D.R.: Consumer health information seeking as hypothesis testing. J. Am. Med. Inform. Assoc. **15**(4), 484–495 (2008)
5. Luo, G., Tang, C., Yang, H., Wei, X.: MedSearch: A specialized search engine for medical information retrieval. In: Proceedings CIKM 2008 (2008)
6. Alfano, M., Lenzitti, B., Taibi, D., Helfert, M.: Facilitating access to health web pages with different language complexity levels. In: Proceedings of the 5th International Conference on Information and Communication Technologies for Ageing Well and e-Health. ICT4AWE, vol. 1, pp. 113–123 (2019). https://doi.org/10.5220/0007740301130123. ISBN 978-989-758-368-1
7. Kummervold, E., Chronaki, C.E., Lausen, B., Prokosch, H.U.: A population based survey. J. Med. Internet Res. **10**, 42 (2008)

8. Instituto Nacional de Estadística: Encuesta sobre Equipamiento y Uso de Tecnologías de la Información y Comunicación en los hogares (2010)

9. UK National Statistics: Statistical bulletin: Internet Access 2010. Office for National Statistics (2010). Accessed 27 Aug 2010

10. Pletneva, N., Vargas, A., Boyer, C.: Requirements for the general public health search. Khresmoi Publ. Deliv. **D8**(1), 1 (2011)

11. Keselman, A., Slaughter, L.: Towards consumer-friendly PHRs: patients' experience with reviewing their health records. In: AMIA Annual Symposium Proceedings, pp. 399–403 (2007)

12. Alfano, M., Lenzitti, B., Taibi, D., Helfert, M.: Provision of tailored health information for patient empowerment: an initial study. In: CompSysTech 2019: 20-th International Conference on Computer Systems and Technologies, University of Ruse, Bulgaria, 21–22 June 2019. ACM, New York (2019)

13. Banna, S., Hasan, H., Dawson, P.: Understanding the diversity of user requirements for interactive online health services. Int. J. Healthc. Technol. Manag. **15**(3), 253–271 (2016)

14. Roberts, T.: Searching the Internet for health information: techniques for patients to effectively search both public and professional websites. In: SLE Workshop at Hospital for Special Surgery Tips For Evaluating the Quality of Health, pp. 1–12 (2017)

15. Pian, W., Khoo, C.S.G., Chi, J.: Automatic classification of users' health information need context: logistic regression analysis of mouse-click and eye-tracker data. J. Med. Internet Res. **19**(12), e424 (2017)

16. Pang, P. C.-I., Verspoor, K., Pearce, J., Chang, S.: Better health explorer: designing for health information seekers. In: OzCHI 2015 Proceedings of the Annual Meeting of the Australian Special Interest Group for Computer Human Interaction, pp. 588–597 (2015). https://doi.org/10.1145/2838739.2838772

17. Keselman, A., Logan, R., Smith, C.: Developing informatics tools and strategies for consumer-centered health communication. J. Am. Med. Inf. Assoc.: JAMIA **15**(4), 473–483 (2008). https://doi.org/10.1197/jamia.M2744

18. Ardito, S.C.: Seeking consumer health information on the Internet **37**(4) 1–5 (2013). http://www.infotoday.com/OnlineSearcher/Articles/Medical-Digital/Seeking-Consumer-Health-Information-on-the-Internet-90558.shtml

19. Alfano, M., Lenzitti, B., Lo Bosco, G., Perticone, V.: An automatic system for helping health consumers to understand medical texts. In: Proceedings of HEALTHINF 2015, Lisbon, pp. 622–627 (2015)

20. Alfano, M., Lenzitti, B., Lo Bosco, G., Taibi, D.: Development and practical use of a medical vocabulary-thesaurus-dictionary for patient empowerment. In: Proceedings of ACM International Conference on Computer Systems and Technologies (CompSysTech 2018), Ruse (2018)

21. Dietze, S., Taibi, D., Yu, R., Barker, P., d'Aquin M.: Analysing and improving embedded markup of learning resources on the Web. In: Proceedings of the 26th International Conference on World Wide Web Companion (WWW 2017 Companion), pp. 283–292, International World Wide Web Conferences Steering Committee, Republic and Canton of Geneva, Switzerland (2017). https://doi.org/10.1145/3041021.3054160

22. Taibi, D., Fetahu, B., Dietze, S.: Towards integration of Web data into a coherent educational data graph. In: WWW 2013 Companion - Proceedings of the 22nd International Conference on World Wide Web, pp. 419–424 (2013)

23. Meusel, R., Petrovski, P., Bizer, C.: The WebDataCommons microdata, RDFa and microformat dataset series. In: Mika, P., Tudorache, T., Bernstein, A., Welty, C., Knoblock, C., Vrandečić, D., Groth, P., Noy, N., Janowicz, K., Goble, C. (eds.) ISWC 2014. LNCS, vol. 8796, pp. 277–292. Springer, Cham (2014). https://doi.org/10.1007/978-3-319-11964-9_18

24. Kloehn, N., et al.: Improving consumer understanding of medical text: Development and validation of a new subsimplify algorithm to automatically generate term explanations in English and Spanish. J. Med. Internet Res. **20**(8), e10779 (2018)
25. Leroy, G., et al.: Improving perceived and actual text difficulty for health information consumers using semi-automated methods. In: AMIA Annual Symposium Proceedings, pp. 522–531 (2012)
26. Alfano, Marco, Lenzitti, Biagio, Taibi, Davide, Helfert, Markus: ULearn: personalized medical learning on the web for patient empowerment. In: Herzog, Michael A., Kubincová, Zuzana, Han, Peng, Temperini, Marco (eds.) ICWL 2019. LNCS, vol. 11841, pp. 217–228. Springer, Cham (2019). https://doi.org/10.1007/978-3-030-35758-0_20
27. Alfano, M., Lenzitti, B., Lo Bosco, G.: U-MedSearch: a meta search engine of medical content for different users and learning needs. In: Proceedings of International Conference on e-Learning (e-Learning 2015), Berlin (2015)
28. Alfano, M., Lenzitti, B., Lo Bosco, G.: A Web search methodology for health consumers. In: Proceedings of ACM International Conference on Computer Systems and Technologies (CompSysTech 2014), pp. 150–157, Ruse (2014)

Participatory Design of Historytelling Voice Assistance with Older Adults

Torben Volkmann$^{(\boxtimes)}$, Michael Sengpiel, Rita Karam, and Nicole Jochems

Universität zu Lübeck, Ratzeburger Allee 160, 23562 Lübeck, Germany
{volkmann,sengpiel,karam,jochems}@imis.uni-luebeck.de

Abstract. Using information and communication technology (ICT) becomes increasingly important for older adults, yet designers often fail to develop usable software for this group, creating a strong incentive to include older adults in a participatory development process. This paper describes how older adults have been included throughout the development process of a storytelling input component for the Historytelling (HT) project, to attain the best possible usability for older adults. HT provides a digital interactive platform for older adults to share life stories across generations, potentially improving their health and well-being and follows the HCD+ (Human Centered Design for Aging) approach. 19 older adults (M = 68 years old) participated in three studies to analyze, evaluate and design a storytelling voice assistance including a conversational agent. They contributed substantially to the development of the HT project by their involvement in the design process with methods adjusted to comprise characteristics of older adults, addressing three central research questions regarding the type of voice input suitable for older adults, the minimal requirements for a conversational agent and the design of a suitable dialogue system.

Keywords: Human-centered design for aging · Participatory design · Voice user interface

1 Introduction

With the demographic change, the percentage of older adults steadily increases, while new information and communication technology (ICT) emerges at an ever faster pace. To attain the best possible usability for older adults, it has become imperative to include them in the development process and value them as possible co-designers [32], for who would know better about their needs and desires?

The Historytelling project (HT) is a research project building on the strengths of older adults, providing a tool to tell their life stories on a digital platform and to share them with other people. HT seeks to have a positive influence on three levels: (1) On the societal level, HT fosters multi-perspective historiography, (2) on the group level it strengthens family bonds and friendships, and (3) on the individual level it provides a place to actively reminisce

© Springer Nature Switzerland AG 2020
M. Ziefle and L. A. Maciaszek (Eds.): ICT4AWE 2019, CCIS 1219, pp. 101–118, 2020.
https://doi.org/10.1007/978-3-030-52677-1_6

and reach out to others. The HT-project addresses these levels with a digital social platform specifically designed for and with older adults, giving them the power to record, visualize and share their life stories.

One key aspect of HT is the actual storytelling, for which speech seems to be the most natural channel, since stories are mostly passed on in face to face conversations, which have potentially positive effects on the listeners [2,15, 43]. Transferring this conversational element to technology in the best manner possible is a particular challenge for the HT project.

Alongside the development of a voice component for HT, three research questions were explored: (Q1) Which type of voice input is suitable for older adults? (Q2) What are minimal requirements for a conversational agent for older adults in the context of Historytelling? (Q3) How could the conversational agent dialogue be designed?[1] To answer these research questions and develop the actual HT with voice input, we followed the HCD+ (Human Centered Design for Aging) approach, focusing on participatory design and consideration of user characteristics [32], and including older adults throughout the development process.

1.1 Voice Communication Technology

Schafer [30] as well as Cohen and Oviatt [5] specify advantages of voice input: it is the natural way to communicate; it is usable even if the hands or eyes are busy; it is accessible for handicapped people; sometimes natural language interaction is preferred and "pronunciation is the subject matter of computer use" [5].

Schafer [30] also lists four challenges regarding voice communication technology: (1) hardware/software implementation of the system, (2) synthesis for voice output, (3) speech recognition and understanding voice input, and (4) usability factors related to how humans interact with machines.

Digital voice assistants such as Amazon Echo, Google Home and Apple Siri have recently been developed and marketed to increase the overall usage of voice input systems. Insofar, the longstanding problem of speech recognition and understanding of voice input has been solved for the consumer market, at least in a narrow context [13,14,20] and new developments of neural networks keep improving voice recognition [1].

Technologically, there are three options to handle voice input: audio recording, speech-to-text processing and automatic transcription. Audio recording is possible using various ICT, such as laptops, tablets and smartphones. Speech-to-text processing converts spoken words instantaneously into text, whereas the automatic transcription converts the recorded audio to text afterwards and is often used for automatic interview transcription.

---

[1] The first two questions have already been addressed in the conference proceeding [41], on which this chapter is largely based. Q3 has been a later addition to the project and reflects our ongoing HT research and development.

1.2 Embodied Conversational Agents

With HTs focus on reminiscing and passing on life stories, users' emotional reactions should be expected and accommodated in the user interface (UI) design. For example, avatars could respond to emotional stories with facial expressions and gestures [35]. Sutcliffe [35] proposes a taxonomy based on 22 emotions, split into reactions to events, agents (other people) and objects to design suitable reactions of systems using the OCC (Ortny, Clore, Collins) model.

Embodied conversational agents (ECA) could integrate these emotions via faces, gaining recent research attention [36]. ECAs are virtual characters having the same properties as humans in face-to-face communication and they have been integrated successfully into projects with older adults [4]. Older adults followed ECAs instructions better than those provided by classic user interfaces and they had a subjectively positive influence in recall tasks [27,37]. Isbister & Doyle [16] developed a taxonomy relevant for the development of an ECA. It consists of five categories to classify and evaluate ECAs: (1) Believability, (2) Social interface, (3) Application domains, (4) Agency and computational issues and (5) Production.

1.3 Cooperative Conversation Principle

Cooperation and dialogue principles play a central role in the design of an embodied conversational agent [9,39], and communication theory can be very useful in the development of computer systems in general, as a symbiosis of these fields can help to enrich and clarify concepts of both [7,25]. Communication research established maxims of communication to describe challenges and general goals in the multiplicity of communication. Especially well-known and useful are the communication maxims of Grice [12], stating that conversations are to some

Table 1. Grice's maxims of the cooperative principle pursuing effective communication.

Maxim	Examples
Quality	– **supermaxim:** "Try to make your contribution one that is true."
	– Do not say what you believe is false
	– Do not say that for which you lack adequate evidence
Quantity	– Make your contribution as informative as is required
	– Do not make your contribution more informative than is required
Relation	– "Be relevant"
Manner	– **supermaxim:** "Be perspicuous."
	– Avoid obscurity of expression
	– Avoid ambiguity
	– Be brief
	– Be orderly

extent purpose-oriented, are based on cooperative efforts and consist of discon-nected remarks where each participants recognizes a "mutually accepted direc-tion". They are divided into four maxims shown in Table 1: (1) quantity, (2) quality, (3) relation and (4) manner. These maxims can guide the behavior of conversation partners and contribute to a purposeful conversation.

1.4   Participatory Design Process

Participatory design is often seen as a third space of human computer interac-tion, combining different stakeholders' (e.g. user and developer) knowledge to attain new insights and perform new actions [23]. Participatory design involves prospective users in a discussion about functionality, features or look-and-feel of a future product to support fundamental design decisions. It is particularly useful if the developers are not specialists in the observed field. Involving older adults in participatory design creates special demands on the methods. Some conventional design methods may even be inappropriate for them [10].

For HT-development, the HCD+ approach [32] was used, emphasizing the importance of involving users in every critical design step. HCD+ also provides guidelines regarding the recruitment of participants, the atmosphere when work-ing with older adults and required adaptations concerning the concrete execution of methods.

Orso et al. [26] found in a literature review, that especially the following methods are used when older adults are involved in designing interactive tech-nology: (1) visual prompts (graphical representation of an abstract concept), (2) experiencing (giving a direct first-person perspective, i.e. with video sketches), (3) hands on (evoking the reaction and opinion on a tool by providing a physical object instead of a conceptual prototype) and (4) natural tasks (performing a task that is similar to the final context of use).

This paper describes the process of developing a storytelling input compo-nent. Thus, older adults tested and evaluated current technological approaches in the analysis phase. An experimental game was conducted to develop specific design elements in the design and conception phase, a conversational agent's dia-logue sequence was developed and finally, a task-based evaluation of the devel-oped interface was conducted.

2   Voice Input Analysis

2.1   Method

State-of-the-art software was reviewed to answer the first research question ("Which type of voice input is suitable for older adults?"), focusing on the three different input technologies. In the initial study, a task-based evaluation was conducted due to the potential lack of computer literacy among older adults [6,31]. Particularly in the beginning [44], interviews are an important method in the HCD process.

Eight older adults, four men and four women, aged between 60 and 73 ($M = 67.5$, $SD = 3.7$) participated in the evaluation. They were recruited through personal contacts, mailing lists and notice boards. Seven interviews took place at the university, and one at home due to physical handicap.

The evaluation comprised three parts: (1) In the introduction, participants introduced themselves and were asked about key aspects of their life and technology usage. (2) In the practical work phase, participants solved tasks using three different input approaches. "Google docs" was used to demonstrate the speech-to-text capabilities and the software "Speak a Message" was used for audio recording and transcription. Qualitative post-interviews were conducted after every task. (3) As a follow-up, participants were asked for their favorite input approach and filled in a questionnaire testing their computer literacy [31] and affinity for technology [11].

2.2   Results

All participants stated that an assistance system and better feedback by the software would be appreciated. Since feedback preferences varied, visual and auditory assistance should be combined. In particular, participants knew little about current audio transcription methods and technical capabilities and were positively surprised about the initial quality of the automatic transcription.

Participants' computer literacy and affinity towards technology varied greatly. While some participants were confident using the presented software, others needed more time to adjust to the tasks. Faster participants showed a higher computer literacy and affinity towards technology and stated that they tend to find solutions on their own when problems occur.

All ($N = 8$) participants had either a laptop (6) or a computer (3) at home and used either a smartphone (5) or a cell phone (3). They used computers for an average of 19 hours ($SD = 7$) per week, mainly for word processing, emailing and targeted information search. They scored an average of $M = 20.4$ ($SD = 4.17$) on the computer literacy scale (CLS, max $= 26$), which is low compared to a younger group ($M = 23.9$), but high compared to other older adults ($M = 14.4$, [31]). Also, they scored an average of $M = 2.8$ on the affinity for technology interaction scale (ATI, $SD = 0.9$, scale ranging from 1 to 6).

Participants. Participants stated that their technical difficulties were situational and rather hard to describe. When problems occurred, they would mainly turn to friends or family or seek professional help. Three participants stated they would first try to find the solution on their own, yet they also desired assistance provided by the device itself. Alternatively, integrated tutorials as videos would be appreciated, an approach that has been described by Sengpiel & Wandke [33] among others. The practical part of the study was conducted with 7 of the 8 participants.

Speech-to-Text. Five of the seven participants had never used speech-to-text input, and even the two participants who had used this technology before were surprised by the accuracy of the results. Three participants declared that the conversion from speech to text was too slow, impairing oral fluency. Also, some problems with speech were ambiguous and in some cases problems were not noticed by the participants at all. The software was not "user friendly", since finding functionality was difficult and it was not clear when the recording had started.

Speech-to-Audio. Six of the seven participants had used a dictation device to record audio before. Most notably, they liked the simplicity of dictation, the option to replay and edit recordings later, and the authentically captured audio atmosphere.

Transcription. No participant had used audio transcription before, but five out of seven participants liked the option to have both, audio and text. The unobtrusiveness of the method was particularly well received, for it allowed to maintain oral fluency. Even so, the quality of the initial transcription was crucial for further adoption.

Preferred Input Method. Participants' method preferences were largely influenced by overall quality and usability aspects, while intended audience and purpose were key drivers as well. If the goal was to quickly write a short story, participants chose the speech-to-text input. The transcription technology was preferred for longer, more meaningful stories. Table 2 shows the frequencies of acceptance with participants indicating acceptance for one or more methods. Since older adults preferred the transcription technology, it will be used for further development.

Table 2. Frequencies of indicated acceptance for one or more input methods ($N = 8$).

Technology	Frequency of acceptance
Transcription	6
Audio recording	2
Speech-to-text	4

3   Age-Appropriate Design

3.1   Method

To address the second research question ("What are minimal requirements for a conversational agent for older adults in the context of Historytelling?"), a

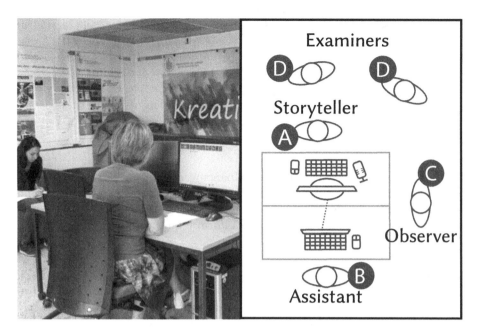

Fig. 1. Photograph and sketch of the simulation game's setup; A = Storyteller, B = Assistant, C = Observer, D = Examiner.

workshop with three different groups was conducted. Since participants were expected to have lower computer literacy, technology was partly replaced by a real-life example (see also [21,32]).

There are a variety of methods using real life examples as prototypes for technology development, among them "invisible technology videos" [21], (Cultural) Probes [3], and Forum Theater [29]. We used a simulation game often used in educational context, more specifically a modified simulation game used by Reich [18]. He states that the ideal simulation game consists of seven phases: (1) introduction, (2) information and reading, (3) opinion-forming and strategy planning, (4) interaction within the groups, (5) preparation of a plenum, (6) conducting a plenum, (7) game evaluation. To save time in the workshop, the phases two and three were removed and conducted by the researchers beforehand, while phase seven was conducted by the researchers after the workshop. Nine older women (M = 68) were recruited as participants through the "Deutscher Frauenring e.V.", a leading women's organization in Germany. They took part in three rounds within a larger full day workshop with multiple parts on the University campus. A desktop microphone and the software "Speak a Message" running on a laptop with external screen and mouse was used to record their interactions.

The simulation game lasted 15 min per round and was followed by seven minutes for discussion. Then, participants were interviewed according to their respective roles: (A) Storyteller: *"Please read aloud this shortened version of "Mother Hulda". The assistant will help you with the recording."* (B) Assistant: *"Please simulate a voice assistant. Remain within your role and react to anything you notice."* (C) Observer: *"Please observe the interaction between the assistant and the storyteller and fill in this observation sheet."* The storyteller and the assistant were positioned to have no direct eye contact, while the observer was asked to sit seeing both, assistant and storyteller, as shown in Fig. 1.

3.2   Results

The simulation game revealed that participants were good at taking perspective, eager to provide meaningful information and help with their expertise and had no problems solving the tasks given. In the follow-ups there were lively discussions about possible improvements, which will inform requirements for the assistance system.

Participants. All nine older adults aged between 57 and 77 (M = 68.3, SD = 5,1) were women. They all owned a smartphone and seven used it frequently. Also, eight of them used their computer or laptop frequently, mostly for communication and targeted information search. As expected for their age group, they scored relatively low on the computer literacy scale (CLS: M = 16, SD = 3.67) but (unexpectedly) high on the affinity for technology scale (ATI: M = 3.8, SD = 0.8).

Simulation Game. Simulation game results are quite diverse between groups, showing very different behavior. For example, group 2 had a fluent dialogue, while the other groups had rather functional dialogues, e.g.:

Group 2: Assistant: *"I am the voice assistant. My name is..."* Storyteller: *"I am the storyteller. My name is... and I will start right away."*

Groups 1 & 3: Assistant: *"I am the voice assistant. My name is... Have you turned on your microphone?"* Storyteller: *"Yes, should I press the record button?"* Assistant: *"Yes"*

Group 1 did not establish a fluent dialogue, yet in the interview the storyteller said she would have liked a more fluent dialogue and better feedback from the assistant, especially regarding recording quality.

Group 2 established a fluent dialogue from the start and immediately reacted to the assistant's remark to speak louder. However, in the interview the storyteller considered this interruption unpleasant and said she would prefer visual help and remarks, for any interruption in the flow of storytelling should be avoided.

Group 3 started with a longer dialogue, but the storyteller had forgotten to record it. The assistant said in the interview that she had noticed it, but did not want to interrupt the storyteller, conceding afterwards that it would have been better to do so. They also appreciated the dialogue in the beginning and wished it could have been continued in the study as well as with the technical system to be developed.

Resulting Interface Requirements. Based on the simulation game, some requirements were developed for the assistance system: It should answer user questions with a fluent verbal dialogue, being able to assess events' relevance and adapt kind and timing of communication to avoid unnecessary interruptions. In essence, the participants hoped for an assistance system behaving like a polite competent human, perhaps pushing the boundaries of today's technology. Especially the recording flow should be supported from start to finish. There are further requirements for voice input communication in the literature, some of which were pointed out in Sect. 1.1.

3.3 Resulting Interface

The resulting high-fidelity prototype is based on an interface published in a 2019 paper [40] to ensure consistency within the HT project. Since the prototype could not display dynamic content, interface elements had to remain static. Thus, some interactions such as providing feedback in recording sessions were triggered by the experimenter as Wizard of Oz. There were four kinds of feedback:

- Visualization based on a VU (volume units) meter (a standard display for the signal level in audio equipment, see Fig. 2 top left).
- Warning messages (see Fig. 2 bottom).
- An earcon (ear + icon [34], which are "abstract, synthetic and mostly musical tones or sound patterns that can be used in structured combination" [8]).
- A voice assistant in form of an ECA as described in Sect. 1.2 (see Fig. 2 top right).

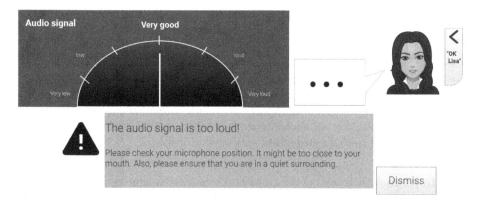

Fig. 2. Interface elements of the prototype developed. top left: VU meter used for audio visualization, top right: Voice assistant Lisa speaking, bottom: warning message.

Assistance is provided in three standardized, consecutive steps. First, a problem in audio quality is visualized through the VU meter. If the user does not perceive the problem and thus cannot deal with it, an earcon was played and an additional warning message displayed, announcing that the recording will be stopped. For the last step, the assistance varied. First there was no additional warning. In a second implementation, an avatar gave information about the problem.

4   Dialogue Design

4.1   Method

To address the third research question on how a conversational agent's dialogue could be designed, a Hierarchical Task Analysis (HTA) regarding the story creation process of the Historytelling project was conducted. The (spoken) dialogue integrates all Historytelling components, assisting users in every step of the (hi)storytelling process. HTA helps to visualize the various tasks and to derive individual dialogue steps (see Fig. 3). From the HTA, three main aspects emerged: (1) The user should be greeted by name. If the name is unknown, it should be asked for to improve personalization of the assistant. (2) The assistant should ask if the user wants to write or read a story. (3) If the user wants to write a new story, the assistant should guide the user through the story creation process described on the bottom of Fig. 3.

Additional challenges for the agent include older adults' difficulties to remember details of their life stories while telling them. Naturally, the stories could also trigger various (intense) emotions, necessitating adequate reactions from the agent. These challenges have to be taken into account when developing the dialogue system, which should also be evaluated based on the cooperative conversation principle.

4.2   Results

Based on the HTA, a dialogue sequence was developed bearing Paul Grice's principles of conversation [12] in mind, aiming to support older adults telling their life stories. It consists of 29 items in multiple branches, creating the impression of a conversation in natural language. First, a non-embodied chatbot was developed, that will later be enhanced to an embodied virtual agent. Items of the dialogue sequence can be categorized as shown in Table 3.

First Implementation. The first prototype of the dialogue system was implemented based on web technologies. Its basic system model is shown in Fig. 4. Mozilla Web Speech API [22] was used for automatic speech recognition and speech synthesis via text-to-speech. Natural language understanding and generation were implemented using RiveScript [28], a scripting language developed for chatbots. First tests with the user group showed that response times were often too high and the designed dialogue sequence has to be improved iteratively.

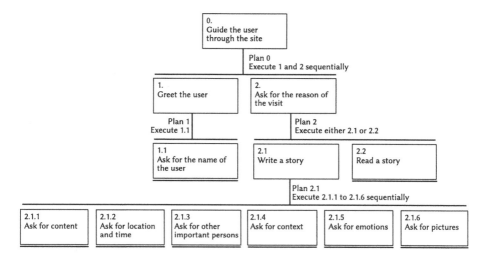

Fig. 3. Hierarchical Task Analysis (HTA) for a conversational agent's dialogue.

Table 3. Categorized items of the conversational agent's dialogue sequence.

Purpose	Explanation	Example
Greet the user	The user is greeted to show that a dialogue can be started. The assistant introduces himself and may ask for the user's name	"Welcome, I am your personal assistant. What is your name?"
Ask for purpose of visit	If the user wants to read stories, stories will be suggested. Otherwise, the storytelling process begins	"It is nice having you here! Would you like to tell a story?"; "Great! What do you want to talk about?"
Support remembering	The assistant may help with remembering parts of a story or helps with starting to narrate	"That is no problem. Then just let us think together"
Support the story creation	The assistant supports the process of describing the story	"Very good! You can add the location by clicking on the marker symbol. Just search for the location and click on linking."
Help to enrich the content	The assistant may encourage the user, to write a meaningful and vivid story	"I am very happy about that and I am sure that your listeners will like it as well"

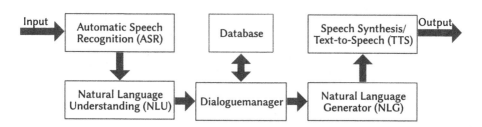

Fig. 4. Basic system model of the dialogue system; based on [17].

5   Evaluation

To assess usability and user experience of the interface, a Wizard of Oz evaluation was conducted, where participants had to record a story with the provided interface and assistance as described in Sect. 3.3. Two questions were essential for this evaluation: (1) Has the assistance been perceived? (2) Which assistance was preferred?

Eight older adults aged between 61 and 70 years (M = 66, SD = 3) took part in the evaluation, five of them were male and three female, and six had already participated in the first study. They were recruited through personal contacts, mailing lists and notice boards.

All evaluations took place at the university. A Christmas flower and a candle were placed around the participants and cake, water and hot drinks were served [24] to create a comfortable atmosphere.

Figure 5 shows part of the room in which the evaluation was conducted. Behind the participant (A), the wizard (B) and the recorder (C) were present in the room. First, participants received questionnaires regarding demographic information, affinity for technology [11] and computer literacy [31]. Then, the participants used the voice input interface with randomized order of assistance interface. Before each run, the microphone was secretly placed too far from the participants, causing a problem with audio quality, to justify the system warning and trigger a response from the participants. Before the run of the classic interface, the microphone cable was unplugged as well. After the recorded interaction with the user interface, participants filled out the User Experience Questionnaire (UEQ [19]). The second interface was tested accordingly. Lastly, adjustment options and preferred interfaces were discussed in an interview.

5.1   Results

Overall, the Wizard of Oz prototype proved useful to test functionality that would have been difficult to implement, such as the transcription or the avatar. The simple prototype allowed for participants' immersion in the storytelling process, although wizard response time was sometimes too high to satisfy participants.

Participants. The eight older participants aged 61 to 70 years (M = 66, SD = 3, five women and three men), mainly used computers, tablets and smart phones, mostly for text editing, email, internet searching and surfing. Considering their age, they had relatively high computer literacy (CLS: M = 21.8, SD = 4.1) and high affinity for technology (ATI: M = 3.1, SD = 1.1).

Awareness of Provided Feedback. All participants perceived the information provided by the voice assistant about occurring problems, but they did not engage in conversation. They used the provided VU meter for regular monitoring, yet the earcon was often ignored or not perceived at first, especially by those

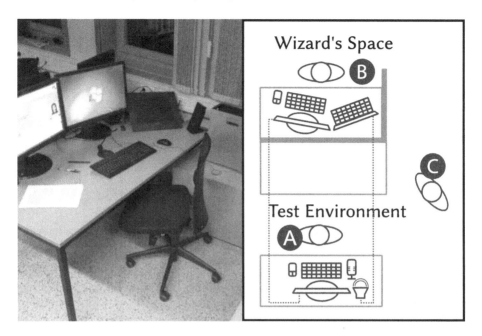

Fig. 5. Photograph and sketch of the evaluation setup; based on [41].

immersed in storytelling. Only three of eight participants perceived the earcon from the start, three more perceived it the second time. It seems that earcons need to be learnt before use [8]. A combined approach considering the importance of the intervention might work best in this scenario. Giving the storyteller information how to improve the quality of the audio signal, while maintaining oral fluency of the storytelling process, seems to be very challenging.

Preferred Assistance. The User Experience Questionnaire (UEQ) revealed a strong preference for voice assistance, but only if feedback was triggered on time. If it was delayed, then discomfort, confusion, and frustration occurred, and participants rated the User Experience much lower in all UEQ categories. However, delays had much smaller impact on the UEQ score when the interface was used without voice assistant. Figure 6 shows this interaction effect for voice assistant x delay based on UEQ mean scores across the scales found in Table 4.

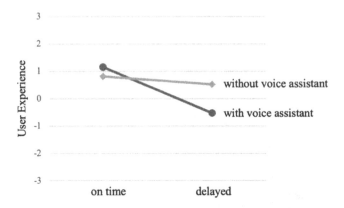

Fig. 6. Interaction effect for voice assistant x delay on User Experience Questionnaire (UEQ) mean scores (see Table 4 for details); see [41].

Table 4. Results of the User Experience Questionnaire (Scale ranging from −3 to +3) for recordings with and without voice assistant, either delayed or on time, indicating an interaction effect also seen in Fig. 6.

Aspect	Recordings with voice assistant				Recordings without voice assistant			
	On time (N = 5)		Delayed (N = 3)		On time (N = 5)		Delayed (N = 3)	
	M	SD	M	SD	M	SD	M	SD
Attractiveness	1.4	1.1	−0.7	0.8	0.8	1.0	0.3	1.0
Perspicuity	1.5	0.8	−1.2	0.6	1.3	1.3	1.0	0.9
Efficiency	1.3	0.7	−0.3	0.3	1.0	0.8	1.0	0.7
Dependability	0.8	0.8	−1.2	0.4	0.4	1.3	0.5	1.1
Stimulation	1.2	0.5	0	0.8	1.0	1.3	0.3	1.2
Novelty	0.9	0.6	0.2	0.7	0.7	0.4	0.0	1.0
Mean	1.2		−0.5		0.8		0.5	

6   Discussion

In a participatory design project for the Historytelling system, older adults were integrated as potential users in all steps of development of the voice input component and methods were adjusted to accommodate their user characteristics as described in the HCD+ approach [32]. Even though the older study participants scored comparatively high on the computer literacy scale, there was also large heterogeneity within the group, which shows that age as sole indicator for recruiting is not sufficient and questionnaires such as the CLS [31] should be considered to categorize participants. Overall, the adjustments made for including older adults proved beneficial toward the goal of universal usability not to exclude anyone by design. Through the adaptation and method selection, we have managed to create a vibrant atmosphere and engaged the participants in lively discussions which fostered a wide range of results.

Addressing the first research question "Which type of voice input is suitable for older adults", the subsequent transcription was preferred among participants, as they wanted to have both, text and recorded audio. Sadly, there were many errors in the transcript, since the quality of the text to speech engine used in the tested software was not sufficient to maintain uninterrupted oral fluency. To assess the acceptable fault tolerance, additional studies have to be conducted and it remains to be seen if current technology can attain it. Until then, we suggest weighing its potential benefits to the loss in user experience due to frustration.

Addressing the second research question on minimal requirements for a conversational agent for older adults in the context of HT, users should be guided through the recording process. A virtual speech assistant giving necessary information could be helpful, but it should recede into the background during story recording and graphical user interface elements should be used for regular monitoring instead. The evaluation has shown that the assistance provided as Wizard of Oz prototype was immersive, but a delay in the assistants' feedback should be avoided, because it cripples user experience, upending the benefits of conversational agents and leaving the users uncomfortable and confused. Moreover, users faced with the virtual speech assistant prototype acted differently than those faced with the simulation game used for requirement analysis. With the prototype, users concentrated more on story telling, whereas the simulation often provoked real conversations between human story teller and human voice assistant.

For practical application, the HT system could (continuously) monitor whether voice assistance can be delivered without noticeable delay (e.g. due to low available bandwidth, bad sound input quality, noisy surroundings or users speaking too softly), and conceal it otherwise to avoid the "UX penalty" for a delayed voice assistant shown in Fig. 6 and Table 4. However, this could also necessitate a removal of such functionality, which could in itself be more frustrating to the user than not knowing a voice assistant existed. To alleviate such frustration, the HT system would need to communicate the reasons to the user transparently and comprehensibly. Also, audio files could be stored and transcribed later (with enhanced technology). In the HT context, volunteers might also be willing to correct errors in the transcripts for the storytellers.

Regarding the third research question on how a conversational agent's dialogue could be designed, it became apparent that a combination of graphical user interface and voice user interfaces could address the needs of older adults— a combined approach is not yet supported in commercial products such as Alexa and Siri, but has been investigated in research projects including our own and seems very promising especially for older users.

Finally, privacy concerns play an important role in technology acceptance and adoption, especially for older users. For that reason, cloud based commercial systems such as Alexa and Siri may not be suitable for them and could eventually be replaced by alternatives such as Mozilla Web Speech. Future HT development and research will also investigate the combination of graphical and voice interfaces and extend the already established style guide [42]. As HT development continues, our progress will be published on the project website [38] and in future publications.

References

1. Arik, S.O., et al.: Deep voice: real-time neural text-to-speech. In: Proceedings of the 34th International Conference on Machine Learning, vol. 70, pp. 195–204. JMLR.org (2017). http://dl.acm.org/citation.cfm?id=3305381.3305402
2. Bornat, J.: Reminiscence and oral history: parallel universes or shared endeavour? Ageing Soc. **21**(02), 219–241 (2001). https://doi.org/10.1017/S0144686X01008157
3. Brandt, E., Grunnet, C.: Evoking the future: drama and props in user centered design. In: Proceedings of Participatory Design Conference, PDC 2000, pp. 11–20 (2000)
4. Cassell, J.: Embodied conversational interface agents. Commun. ACM **43**(4), 70–78 (2000)
5. Cohen, P.R., Oviatt, S.L.: The role of voice input for human-machine communication. Proc. Natl. Acad. Sci. **92**(22), 9921–9927 (1995)
6. Czaja, S.J., Boot, W.R., Charness, N., Rogers, W.A.: Designing for Older Adults: Principles and Creative Human Factors Approaches, 3rd edn. CRC Press, Boca Raton (2019)
7. De Souza, C.S.: The Semiotic Engineering of Human-Computer Interaction. MIT Press, Cambridge (2005)
8. Dingler, T., Lindsay, J., Walker, B.N.: Learnability of sound cues for environmental features: auditory icons, earcons, spearcons, and speech. International Community for Auditory Display (2008)
9. Dybkjær, L., Bernsen, N.O., Dybkjær, H.: Grice incorporated: cooperativity in spoken dialogue. In: Proceedings of the 16th Conference on Computational Linguistics - Volume 1, COLING 1996, pp. 328–333. Association for Computational Linguistics, Stroudsburg (1996). https://doi.org/10.3115/992628.992686
10. Eisma, R., Dickinson, A., Goodman, J., Syme, A., Tiwari, L., Newell, A.F.: Early user involvement in the development of information technology-related products for older people. Univ. Access Inf. Soc. **3**(2), 131–140 (2004). https://doi.org/10.1007/s10209-004-0092-z
11. Franke, T., Attig, C., Wessel, D.: A personal resource for technology interaction: development and validation of the affinity for technology interaction (ATI) scale. Int. J. Hum.-Comput. Interact. 1–12 (2018). https://doi.org/10.1080/10447318.2018.1456150
12. Grice, H.P., Cole, P., Morgan, J., et al.: Logic and conversation, pp. 41–58 (1975)
13. Hailpern, J., Karahalios, K., DeThorne, L., Halle, J.: VocSyl: visualizing syllable production for children with ASD and speech delays. In: Proceedings of the 12th International ACM SIGACCESS Conference on Computers and Accessibility, pp. 297–298. ACM (2010)
14. Hazen, T.J., Saenko, K., La, C.H., Glass, J.R.: A segment-based audio-visual speech recognizer: data collection, development, and initial experiments, p. 235. ACM Press (2004). https://doi.org/10.1145/1027933.1027972
15. Isbell, R., Sobol, J., Lindauer, L., Lowrance, A.: The effects of storytelling and story reading on the oral language complexity and story comprehension of young children. Early Child. Educ. J. **32**(3), 157–163 (2004). https://doi.org/10.1023/B:ECEJ.0000048967.94189.a3
16. Isbister, K., Doyle, P.: Design and evaluation of embodied conversational agents: a proposed taxonomy. In: The First International Joint Conference on Autonomous Agents & Multi-Agent Systems (2002)

17. Jacko, J.A.: Human Computer Interaction Handbook: Fundamentals, Evolving Technologies, and Emerging Applications, p. 373. CRC Press, Boca Raton (2012)
18. Kersten Reich: Unterrichtsmethoden im konstruktiven und systemischen methodenpool (2017), http://methodenpool.uni-koeln.de/
19. Laugwitz, B., Held, T., Schrepp, M.: Construction and evaluation of a user experience questionnaire. In: Holzinger, A. (ed.) USAB 2008. LNCS, vol. 5298, pp. 63–76. Springer, Heidelberg (2008). https://doi.org/10.1007/978-3-540-89350-9_6
20. Levin, G., Lieberman, Z.: In-situ speech visualization in real-time interactive installation and performance, p. 7. ACM Press (2004). https://doi.org/10.1145/987657.987659
21. Lindsay, S., Jackson, D., Schofield, G., Olivier, P.: Engaging older people using participatory design. In: Proceedings of the SIGCHI Conference on Human Factors in Computing Systems, CHI 2012, pp. 1199–1208. ACM, New York (2012). https://doi.org/10.1145/2207676.2208570
22. Mozilla Corporation: Web Speech API (2019). https://developer.mozilla.org/en-US/docs/Web/API/Web_Speech_API
23. Muller, M.J.: Participatory design: the third space in HCI. Human-Comput. Interact.: Dev. Process **4235**, 165–185 (2003)
24. Newell, A., Arnott, J., Carmichael, A., Morgan, M.: Methodologies for involving older adults in the design process. In: Stephanidis, C. (ed.) UAHCI 2007. LNCS, vol. 4554, pp. 982–989. Springer, Heidelberg (2007). https://doi.org/10.1007/978-3-540-73279-2_110
25. Nobre, G.F., Touring, A.: Political communicative agents. In: Proceedings of the 6th International Conference on Politics and Information Systems, Technologies and Applications, Orlando (FL), pp. 88–93 (2008)
26. Orso, V., Spagnolli, A., Gamberini, L., Ibañez, F., Fabregat, M.E.: Involving older adults in designing interactive technology: the case of SeniorChannel. In: Proceedings of the 11th Biannual Conference on Italian SIGCHI Chapter, CHItaly 2015, pp. 102–109. ACM, New York (2015). https://doi.org/10.1145/2808435.2808464
27. Ortiz, A., del Puy Carretero, M., Oyarzun, D., Yanguas, J.J., Buiza, C., Gonzalez, M.F., Etxeberria, I.: Elderly users in ambient intelligence: does an avatar improve the interaction? In: Stephanidis, C., Pieper, M. (eds.) UI4ALL 2006. LNCS, vol. 4397, pp. 99–114. Springer, Heidelberg (2007). https://doi.org/10.1007/978-3-540-71025-7_8
28. Petherbridge, N.: Artificial intelligence scripting language (2019). https://www.rivescript.com
29. Rice, M., Newell, A., Morgan, M.: Forum Theatre as a requirements gathering methodology in the design of a home telecommunication system for older adults. Behav. Inf. Technol. **26**(4), 323–331 (2007). https://doi.org/10.1080/01449290601177045
30. Schafer, R.W.: Scientific bases of human-machine communication by voice. Proc. Natl. Acad. Sci. **92**(22), 9914–9920 (1995). https://doi.org/10.1073/pnas.92.22.9914
31. Sengpiel, M., Dittberner, D.: The computer literacy scale (CLS) for older adults-development and validation. In: Mensch & Computer, pp. 7–16 (2008)
32. Sengpiel, M., Volkmann, T., Jochems, N.: Considering older adults throughout the development process - The HCD+ approach. In: Proceedings of the Human Factors and Ergonomics Society Europe Chapter 2018 Annual Conference, Berlin (2019)
33. Sengpiel, M., Wandke, H.: Compensating the effects of age differences in computer literacy on the use of ticket vending machines through minimal video instruction. Occup. Ergon. **9**, 87–98 (2010)

34. Sumikawa, D.: Guidelines for the integration of audio cues into computer user interfaces, June 1985
35. Sutcliffe, A.: Designing user interfaces in emotionally-sensitive applications. In: Bernhaupt, R., Dalvi, G., Joshi, A., K. Balkrishan, D., O'Neill, J., Winckler, M. (eds.) INTERACT 2017. LNCS, vol. 10515, pp. 404–422. Springer, Cham (2017). https://doi.org/10.1007/978-3-319-67687-6_27
36. Tsiourti, C., Joly, E., Wings, C., Moussa, M.B., Wac, K.: Virtual assistive companions for older adults: qualitative field study and design implications. In: Proceedings of the 8th International Conference on Pervasive Computing Technologies for Healthcare, PervasiveHealth 2014, pp. 57–64. ICST (Institute for Computer Sciences, Social-Informatics and Telecommunications Engineering), ICST, Brussels (2014). https://doi.org/10.4108/icst.pervasivehealth.2014.254943
37. Tsiourti, C., Quintas, J., Ben-Moussa, M., Hanke, S., Nijdam, N.A., Konstantas, D.: The CaMeLi framework—A multimodal virtual companion for older adults. In: Bi, Y., Kapoor, S., Bhatia, R. (eds.) IntelliSys 2016. SCI, vol. 751, pp. 196–217. Springer, Cham (2018). https://doi.org/10.1007/978-3-319-69266-1_10
38. Universität zu Lübeck: Historytelling (2019). http://historytelling.eu/
39. Vasardani, M., Timpf, S., Winter, S., Tomko, M.: From descriptions to depictions: a conceptual framework. In: Tenbrink, T., Stell, J., Galton, A., Wood, Z. (eds.) COSIT 2013. LNCS, vol. 8116, pp. 299–319. Springer, Cham (2013). https://doi.org/10.1007/978-3-319-01790-7_17
40. Volkmann, T., Dohse, F., Sengpiel, M., Jochems, N.: Age-appropriate design of an input component for the historytelling project. In: Bagnara, S., Tartaglia, R., Albolino, S., Alexander, T., Fujita, Y. (eds.) IEA 2018. AISC, vol. 822, pp. 672–680. Springer, Cham (2019). https://doi.org/10.1007/978-3-319-96077-7_73
41. Volkmann., T., Sengpiel., M., Karam., R., Jochems., N.: Age-appropriate participatory design of a storytelling voice input in the context of historytelling. In: Proceedings of the 5th International Conference on Information and Communication Technologies for Ageing Well and e-Health - Volume 1: ICT4AWE, pp. 104–112. INSTICC, SciTePress (2019). https://doi.org/10.5220/0007729801040112
42. Volkmann, T., Unger, A., Sengpiel, M., Jochems, N.: Development of an age-appropriate style guide within the historytelling project. In: Zhou, J., Salvendy, G. (eds.) HCII 2019. LNCS, vol. 11592, pp. 84–97. Springer, Cham (2019). https://doi.org/10.1007/978-3-030-22012-9_7
43. Weiss, B., Wechsung, I., Kühnel, C., Möller, S.: Evaluating embodied conversational agents in multimodal interfaces. Comput. Cogn. Sci. 1(1), 1–21 (2015). https://doi.org/10.1186/s40469-015-0006-9
44. Wood, L.E.: Semi-structured interviewing for user-centered design. Interactions 4(2), 48–61 (1997). https://doi.org/10.1145/245129.245134

Development and Evaluation of a Motion-Based Exercise Game for Balance Improvement

Michalis Chartomatsidis and Christos Goumopoulos(✉)

Information and Communication Systems Engineering Department, University of the Aegean, Samos, Greece
icsdd18004@icsd.aegean.gr, goumop@aegean.gr

Abstract. Over the past years many systems involving exercising through games (exergaming) have been developed by leveraging on new technologies to provide an alternative way for improving physical condition and balance control. Such systems are widely used for improving the physical condition of healthy persons and for rehabilitation. For seniors, exergames provide a new and enjoyable way for increasing physical activity and for improving balance condition and muscle strength to reduce fall risks. However, a matter arising is whether such systems are well designed to suit seniors. In this work the development and evaluation of a new exergame is presented. The development process followed a human centered design approach involving the relevant stakeholders to create an effective system for balance training. The implementation was based on the Microsoft Kinect sensor for motion recognition and the Unity graphics engine for creating a realistic three-dimensional open world. The influence of user diversity on gesture training and recognition is discussed and the proper sample size is determined in order to achieve a high confidence level in gestures recognition. Results of a user evaluation study are reported both on balance improvement and on system usability, by using proper measurement instruments. The results indicate a positive acceptance of the technology and the possibility for balance improvement leading to healthier seniors.

Keywords: Motion-based exercise game · Seniors · Microsoft Kinect · Unity engine · Usability evaluation · Balance improvement · Human centered design · Ambient assisted living

1 Introduction

Exercise games (known as exergames) tend to become a useful home-based tool for improving both seniors' physical and mental health by performing game scenario tasks [1]. Furthermore, there is positive evidence that exercise programs that combine balance training and muscle strengthening and coordination can reduce falls and fall risk in the elderly [2].

During the past years off-the-self gaming consoles like Microsoft Kinect XBOX 360, Sony Playstation Eyetoy and Nintendo Wii have been pervasive. Such systems have introduced a new style of physical interaction based on gestures and full body motions

© Springer Nature Switzerland AG 2020
M. Ziefle and L. A. Maciaszek (Eds.): ICT4AWE 2019, CCIS 1219, pp. 119–141, 2020.
https://doi.org/10.1007/978-3-030-52677-1_7

and have been used for training balance and improving fitness for healthy elderly [3] as well as for medical purposes as rehabilitation tools [4].

However, the question that arises is whether such gaming systems that are targeted to the general population following a fit-for-all design approach are appropriate for seniors. Usability studies with the participation of seniors have found that popular commercially available games are not necessarily appropriate for seniors due to their complex interface and game structure [5]. Negative feedback when the players frequently fail to perform game tasks because their movements are slower than expected by the game have been also reported [6]. Many exergames are inappropriate for balance training because they are not properly designed for controlled movements of seniors' body centre of gravity [7] and their use can cause injuries [8]. Furthermore, commercial gaming platforms are not flexible enough to provide exergame personalization taking into account the specific needs of an individual and their cost is considerable.

In this work we introduce the design and development of a game tool that combines Microsoft Kinect technology to capture body movements and gestures and Unity graphics engine to create a 3D semi-opengame world. Moreover we present a human centered design approach for the game mechanics and a set of proper design guidelines that take into account the special needs of seniors. The influence of user diversity on gesture training and recognition is discussed and the proper user sample size for the training process is determined in order to achieve a high confidence level for gestures recognition. The aim was to provide a gaming tool that is both enjoyable to use and has a practical impact on improving seniors balance. To assess the usefulness of the tool a pilot study has been performed with the participation of 12 seniors for a period of five weeks using evaluation metrics such as the Berg Balance Score (BBS), the 30 s sit-to-stand test and validated questionaires for assessing usability factors. The qualitative and quantitative analysis of the pilot data shows that the proposed game tool can be used to assist seniors in improving their balance in an enjoyable and engaging manner. The discussion provides an interpretation of the results and supports the conclusions with evidence from the pilot study and generally accepted knowledge. Future work is outlined regarding the new features to be included in the game and the integration of new technologies to support the future versions of the game tool.

2 Literature Review

The development of computer games for assisting the elderly, mostly for memory training, can be traced back in the 1980s [9]. A new era of research and development initiated when the first tracking sensor, Nintendo Wii was introduced. Later on, the development of Kinect technology introduced a new way of exergaming without the need of holding any controller, making Kinect sensor one of the most viable device for exergaming. These exergames are massively used in the field of Ambient Assisted Living (AAL) as a tool to help elderly remain physically and mentally fit through engaging game activities as well as in the rehabilitation process through specially designed balance exercises [10].

Several studies have explored the appropriateness of commercial game consoles for fall prevention of seniors [11]. In particular the suitability of Microsoft Kinect sensor on enhancing physical exercising and performing rehabilitation protocols has been explored by Mousavi Hondori and Khademi [12]. Their review indicates that Kinect is an adequate device for balance exercising and monitoring of the elderly.

A training intervention program was performed in a nursing home based on the Wii Fit balance board to evaluate the effectiveness of exergaming in reducing the risk of falling in patients with history of falls [13]. Sixty seniors above the age of 65 participated in a six weeks program and received balance training using three balance exergames using body motions while standing on the Wii platform. The study indicated that exergaming can have a positive impact both on physical and psychological well-being assessed through relevant scales the training program provided opportunities for social interactions between the participants when the game was played in groups affecting positively the sense of belonging. A similar study using the Wii balance board was reported in [14]. The study used specially designed exergames and the evaluation showed that using a low cost gaming device and a specially tailored application can be a valid method to assist seniors in improving their well-being and balance self-confidence.

Although the use of commercially available games is promising for the balance training of seniors there is a strong evidence that the development of specially designed games in a process involving all major stakeholders (i.e. elderly, caregivers, physiotherapists and developers) can serve more efficiently exercising intervention goals [15].

A research study performed with elderly in Japan designed and evaluated four exergames developed on the Microsoft Kinect platform with a goal to improve seniors' strength, balance and mobility [16]. The games entailed movements such as grabbing virtual objects using both arms, placing the feet along a straight line, bending knees and hips, crouching and standing on one leg. The users had to perform movements in the context of a game scenario while tasks were becoming more complicated based on the game's level of difficulty. The intervention brought an improvement in daily walking movements as measured by the Berg Balance Scale.

Similar exergames in an AAL environment were examined by Stanmmore et al. [17]. The study focused on whether exergames can be an effective alternative to traditional falls prevention exercise programs for seniors living in sheltered housing. Through a 12-week program which took place in twelve sheltered housing centers, seniors were split into two groups one for standard care and one for standard care including three exergaming sessions per week. The evaluation using the Berg Balance Scale (BBS) showed an increase of 95% in balance due to exergaming.

Studies also are focusing on whether exergaming using consoles can be a helpful tool for patients with chronic diseases. A new exergaming software introduced in [18] called HemoKinect by focusing in patients with hemophilia and evaluating their daily exercise routine using a Kinect V2 sensor. Furthermore, researchers in [19] introduced a three-dimensional exergame based on Kinect sensor for patients with Parkinson's disease. Players interacted with the game using a set of gestures like hitting objects with hands and feet and rotating hip left and right.

The proposed system shares similar goals and embraces the perspective of developing tailored exergames based on a human centered design approach to identify requirements that are closer to the motor and cognitive abilities of seniors. On the sensor technology side, the second version of Microsoft Kinect is used instead of the first one. Besides providing higher resolution, more skeleton joints can be tracked (e.g., thumb joints and hand tip) which allows for identifying more movement combinations. On the game side, further to the basic movements that were used in previous studies, the ability for the user to walk is provided. Moreover, a three-dimensional open world was created using Unity 3D game engine embellished with narrative features through animations, sound and visuals for achieving a more realistic game experience. Although the game requires the use of the Kinect sensor to identify user's movements, there is no dependency on the corresponding game console, thus keeping the cost of the necessary hardware low.

3 Design Methodology

3.1 Human Centered Design

Based on the human centered design (HCD) approach [20] interviews and meetings took place between game designers, seniors and medical experts which allowed for acquiring both qualitative data through brainstorming activities and quantitative data through usability questionnaires to refine the main game characteristics and define the body movements that will be trained throughout the game. Emphasis was given on the motions that were going to be implemented as well as on other game characteristics such as the main game theme. The involvement of seniors under the HCD guidelines from game requirements analysis and design to evaluation was essential in order to adequately capture their preferences and needs.

After every meeting a prototype design was formed using the game ideas exported from the meetings and the mechanisms were evaluated by the users. User feedback on the design and game concepts was analyzed by the users and appropriate changes were implemented. A redesign cycle was followed with refined game rules and interactions before the final prototype development commenced. The iterative user feedback expected to deliver a game tool that will be both useful in terms of balance training and enjoyable in terms of playing experience.

A number of design guidelines for exergames have been gathered by reviewing related research [21] and getting feedback from the elderly people in the HCD process:

- *Body Movements Constraints*: Ageing often leads to both cognitive and physical negative changes, like decline in balance and physical strength. Thus, the game structure must avoid complex movements that may cause injuries. Also, it would be easier for the seniors to deal with only a single task each time.
- *Game Theme*: The theme of the exercise game should be related to real-life activities that are familiar to elderly people. Themes that are associated to natural life such as walking in a forest, picking apples and fishing are more acceptable than artificial settings found in commercial video games.
- *User Interface*: To concentrate on the actual exercise the user interface should be simple and easy to use. All instructions have to be clear and use common language. The interface should have different alternatives for multimedia presentation, such as, text, voice and images. For those who are visually impaired, for example, an audio presentation might be preferable.

- *Provide Instructions*: Learning the game movements before starting the actual game should be provided as a choice to the users. Once those instructions are not required any more, users should have the option to avoid them. Furthermore, it should not be expected that the user will recall the instructions, so every time the user wants to start the game an option to view the instructions should appear.
- *Avoid Small Objects*: It is easier for the elderly to identify large objects rather than small or fast moving.
- *Positive Feedback*: Motivating feedback should be given to encourage play. Constructive feedback should be given to guide and correct exercises. Information and feedback should be given when appropriate, to not disturb the user.
- *Variety of Difficulty Levels*: For users to keep their motivation and continue playing, exergames should include different levels of difficulty. In that way, users will be able to test their skills and try to become better. Also moving to a more difficult level will make users feel that they accomplished something good and the game in fact helps them.

3.2 Game Tool Characteristics

Based on the guidelines mentioned in the previous section a game called "Fruit Collector" was conceptualized. The main purpose of the exergame is to pick up objects that are scattered around the environment and deliver them to appropriate spots. The movements involved in the game design target improvements in balance and walking abilities. Furthermore, other cognitive properties could benefit such as memory, attention and synchronization.

Since the exergame is based on Microsoft Kinect sensor, the game entailed the design of gestures and body movements to interact with the game's environment. Specifically, the game includes the following motions a) Leaning left and right to rotate to the corresponding direction b) on site walking to move forward and c) hand gestures to pick up and drop objects.

During game design the feedback of the user focus group indicated a topic close to the seniors' interests. Thus, the idea was to create a forest with trees and flowers while in the center of it a small village was placed. As for the collected/scattered objects the decision was to be baskets filled with fruits of different types. Finally, the brainstorming indicated that the places to deliver these baskets should be the houses of the village.

Moreover, different levels of difficulty were added to the game. Namely, there are three levels (easy, normal and advanced) and in each level the player must deliver different number of baskets to complete the game; easy requires only two baskets to be delivered, normal requires four baskets and advanced requires the complete set, meaning eight baskets.

A tutorial was added providing simple instructions on how to perform the body movements and how to play the game. Every time the player starts a new game a message is displayed asking whether the player wants to see the tutorial before proceeding on playing.

The game does not provide any negative feedback to the user because as the design guidelines indicated it is important for the seniors to feel confident while playing the game and creating stress and anxiety has to be avoided. On the contrary, when a basket is delivered a positive message is displayed while an appropriate sound is played. After the design process was completed, the game development was progressed in its final phase as will be described in the next section.

4 Kinect Sensor Programming

Microsoft Kinect is a motion tracking sensor based on a depth camera recording technology for skeletal tracking [22] allowing the user to interact with applications using gestures, movements and voice commands without the need to use any controller. For the developed game tool, the second version of the sensor was used (Fig. 1 left) which is equipped with a richer SDK API, the ability to track more joints to identify hand states (Fig. 1 right) and tools to record the motions. Furthermore, the Kinect SDK provides two machine learning algorithms, AdaBoost and Random Forest which can be trained to identify complicated activities. Such activities are recorded using the Visual Gesture Builder tool.

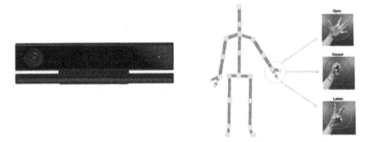

Fig. 1. Left: Kinect Sensor V2, right: Hand states [23].

4.1 Activities Selection and Recording

Besides the motions that already reported above, during the early design stages the game tool included more gestures. Specifically, leaning the head left and right to rotate to the corresponding direction and crouching to move under some obstacles.

Based on the HCD process and interviewing with seniors and domain experts (orthopedics and physiotherapists) the above motions were rejected or modified. Specifically, leaning the head was rejected due to the fact that some seniors had difficulties of a clear view of the game environment while leaning the head, thus this motion was changed to leaning the spine left and right resulting in the same effects. Crouching was also rejected as an interaction motion because of two main reasons. Firstly, the motion was found to be exhaustive and sometimes the reason to quit for many users, and secondly, conflicts occurred with some game scenarios where the user had to crouch and practice on site walking at the same time. As for the on-site walking and the hand gestures no modifications were made.

For game activities recognition a training process was followed by using the recording tool and the machine learning algorithms of the Kinect SDK. For building the activity model the Kinect Studio tool was employed to observe the way the sensor is recording the environment. This tool facilitated also the recording of motions and gestures that were used in the game mechanics. Figure 2 shows, for example, the recording of leaning right and left motions. Such motions are stored in the form of a sequence of frames. A frame is a digitally coded static image represented as a selected number of tracked body parts (i.e. joints). A frame rate of 30 fps (a frame every 0.033 s) was used during activity recording.

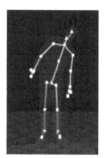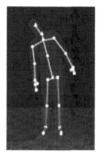

Fig. 2. User leaning right and left.

In order to have more reliable results, the decision was to split the recorded samples into two datasets, one for training and one for validation purposes. In addition, users contributed in recording motions for the training stage did not take part in the final evaluation in order to have more clear results regarding system's ability to identify different users on a variety of motions.

During the training process one issue that required attention was the fact that users cannot execute the movements the same way. Moreover, the body type of each user was an issue that had to be resolved. For instance, some users are taller than others thus, the system would not have been able to identify the gestures and motions if it would have been trained based on a single person.

Furthermore, when it comes to elderly people this issue appears more frequently due to age and physical related issues. Thus, it is expected that the elderly would not perform a specific motion in the same way. For instance, it is expected that seniors would not lean left or right in the same way.

In order to achieve better results regarding the system's ability to identify gestures correctly a group of seniors (male and female) between the age 65 and 70 years with different weight and height characteristics was asked to perform each of the gestures required for game activities. A cycle procedure was followed in order to determine the proper number of users required to train the system to be able to identify the motions with high confidence level. Literature research indicated that the accepted number of people required in situations like this was three in order to cover all body types regarding weight and height. However, after testing that threshold using the live testing option provided by sensor's SDK, it was noticed that system's confidence level was below average. After performing tests with more seniors it was resolved that for the leaning gesture a number of five users is an acceptable limit since the difference in confidence level between 5 and 6 or more users is not significant (Fig. 3).

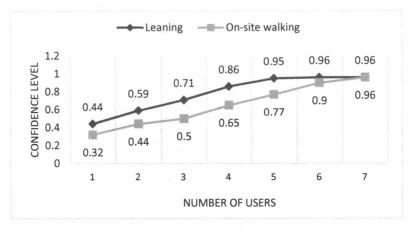

Fig. 3. Average confidence level for each motion in relation to the training user sample.

Regarding the on-site waking motion it turned out to be more a difficult motion for some seniors. Specifically, seniors with less balance control were not able to lift their feet to the same height as others thus requiring more training samples. Therefore, for this type of movement, seven users were found to be the acceptable limit for the training process. Figure 3 shows the confidence level for identifying both gestures in relation to the number of users that participated in the training phase.

4.2 Training Sensor's Algorithm

In order to start the training process, the pre-recorded frame files stored during the recording stage were used. The tuning of the training process entails the selection of several options. These options depend on which parts of the body the sensor will track (upper, lower or both), whether the left and right side of the user's body motion differ and whether the activities are classified as discrete or continuous. A discrete activity is defined as a Boolean entity linked with a confidence value of existence. On the other hand, a continuous activity is associated with a progress value which allows the tool to track its progression optionally via several discrete activities. A continuous activity is more complex, and it is used for motions like dancing or performing certain exercises. The machine learning algorithm that is used for discrete activities is the meta algorithm AdaBoost, whereas for continuous activities the Random Forest algorithm is used. Table 1 shows the selected options for the basic game motions.

As for the walking motion our initial thought was to classify this movement as continuous. A continuous gesture is a combination of two or more discrete gestures and in order to track its progress it has to be split into stages. The user has to pass with success each of these stages for the whole gesture to be successful. In order to split the

Table 1. Options for training gestures [23].

Option	Leaning	Walking
Rely on joints in the lower body	False	True
Rely on hand states	False	False
Right and left side are different	True	True
Discrete/Continuous	Discrete	Discrete

gesture, we use "Tags" to mark the exact timestamp where the user begins to execute the appropriate motion. Figure 4 shows the walking motion split into 5 stages where the pink line indicates the whole gesture and the gray dots are the stages as shown in Table 2.

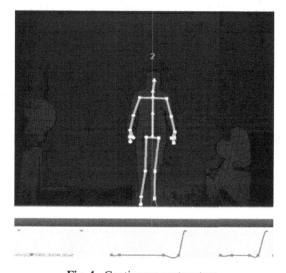

Fig. 4. Continuous gesture tags.

Table 2. Tags for walking gesture.

Stage number	Description
1	User begins to lift left/right foot
2	User begins to lower the raised foot
3	User begins to lift the other foot
4	User begins to lower the raised foot
5	Both feet are on the ground and the gesture is completed

After testing the above scenario, cases were noticed where the system could not recognize the gesture correctly. Specifically, after the end of stage 2 and just before the start of stage 3, the user has both legs on the ground the same as at the end of the gesture which resulted some times in a conflict state, where the system would falsely consider that the motion was completed after stage 2 and right before stage 3. The result of this was for the player to stop moving from time to time which had a negative effect on the overall game experience. Thus, it was decided to reject this approach and classify this motion as discrete and use the same training technique as for the leaning gesture.

The AdaBoost algorithm was used to train the recognition model for leaning and walking motions. After importing the recorded files, the timestamps where the user was performing the corresponding motion were marked. Figure 5 shows the lean left and walking motions performed by a user while the blue lines represent the exact timestamp of that motion.

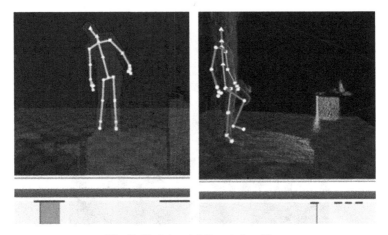

Fig. 5. Training AdaBoost algorithm.

A validation of the trained activity recognition model was performed in order to ensure that the game tool identifies correctly the user's activities. For this purpose, the live testing option was used. Figure 6 shows the tool representation of a senior performing the leaning left motion. The white lines that are passing through the corresponding windows indicate the level of confidence for the gesture.

5   Game Scenery Development

The proposed game tool offers a more realistic game experience than other similar games reported in the literature by playing in a three-dimensional open world. Also, the user is not only limited in executing the game mechanics to complete each level but is also able to explore this game world by executing the same motions described earlier. In this section the steps taken to create the 3D game world are described based on the Unity cross platform game engine.

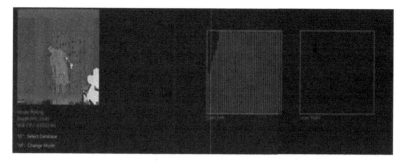

Fig. 6. Validation of leaning left.

The game concept included the creation of a small village inside a forest. Firstly, the terrain on which all the game would take place was created. The terrain's main color is green embellished with some trees and flowers in order to create the forest. At the center of the forest some houses were placed to create the village. Figure 7 illustrates the final view of the village and its textures.

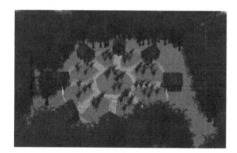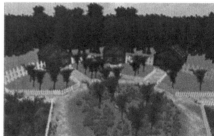

Fig. 7. Game's terrain [23]. (Color figure online)

The game scenery included a number of game objects. Two assets were used to create the baskets and the fruits respectively and by combining these two, one composite game object was created, the basket filled with fruits (Fig. 8). In addition, colors were added to the baskets so that the player can identify them easily. Furthermore, colliders implemented on every game object making the player unable to pass through trees or houses making the game more realistic.

The game also takes advantage of the Unity's particle systems by implementing effects such as explosions or indicators that help the player move forward in the game and improve the whole game experience. Following the HCD design guidelines, indicators were provided in the form of colorful lightning indicators in order for the player to know where to place each basket. Furthermore, these indicators were used in a way of a bonus provider for the player. In particular, if a basket's color was matched to the indicator's the player received double points (Fig. 9). Therefore, players had a motivation to place each basket in the same color spot and so the gaming time could be increased resulting in more user training.

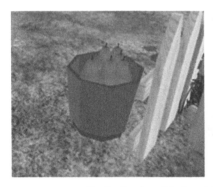 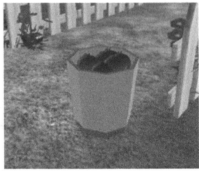

Fig. 8. Baskets filled with fruits. (Color figure online)

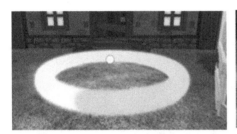 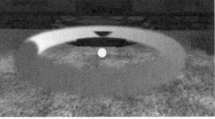

Fig. 9. Lighting indicators. (Color figure online)

An important step was to create the avatar that would be controlled by the user. Unity provides the prefab "First Person character" which has all the utilities needed to complete this task. Furthermore, a target in front of the avatar was added (Fig. 10). The purpose of this was to provide an indication to the player on when the basket could be picked up. Thus, when the avatar is close to the basket the target becomes green otherwise the target remains white.

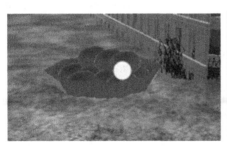 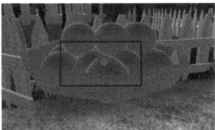

Fig. 10. Target in front of player. (Color figure online)

As for the last step, details that would show the user information about the time and the scoring as well as motivated messages and sounds, which were played when the player completed a task, were added.

5.1 Integration of Kinect with Unity

Microsoft provides a library with various scripts in order to combine Unity projects with the Kinect sensor. The game tool is a combination of scripts from this library, customized scripts created, and C# code added in order to retrieve data from the activities stored during the training stage and to interact with the game.

The flow of control starts with the "Body Source Manager" script which is responsible for activating and deactivating the sensor and tracking the user. This script was customized so that the on-line data from the user's activities are received and processed. Processing is done by the "Activity Detector" script.

Activity Detector receives the output from the "Body Source Manager" script and evaluates it based on the activities included in the AdaBoost's training files. A local database contains all the user's activities required to interact with the game. If the user is performing one of the stored activities a message is sent to "Kinect Manager" script. Kinect Manager receives data indicating if the user is performing a known activity. Specifically, it evaluates the detection confidence and if this is above a defined threshold, it allows the activity to be performed inside the game. For example, if the user is leaning right and the detection confidence is above 60% then the game avatar is rotating to the right.

6 Pilot Study

The evaluation of the game tool took place at the Elderly Protection Center in the city of Ptolemaida, Greece. A group of twelve healthy seniors with an age between 61 and 85 years participated in evaluation study (n = 12, 6 male and 6 females, mean = 73 ± 6.3 years). Once informed consent was obtained the seniors were asked to play the game twice per week for a period of five weeks. In every session each senior was playing the game on all different levels for 25–35 min. The evaluation was organized into four stages and during the whole process a physiotherapist was present for domain-specific support and a researcher for administration and technical support. There were no dropouts.

6.1 Introduction Stage

Firstly, an overview of the technology as well as of the game was given (Fig. 11). The participants received information about the research goals and the scheduled tasks. They were informed about the Kinect device and its applications. From the beginning the seniors showed a great interest in the exergames concept and the supporting technology although they had no relevant experience in the past.

6.2 Physical Condition Assessment

Before the seniors start playing the game, their physical condition was evaluated in order to have a baseline. For this purpose, two widely accepted tests were used: The Berg Balance Scale (BBS) [24] and the 30 s Sit to Stand Test (30SST). The BBS test takes about 15 min and consists of fourteen exercises in order to examine and evaluate

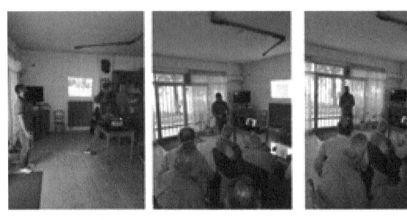

Fig. 11. Seniors learning about the evaluation process [23].

balance control. Examples of the test challenges include (Fig. 12): standing for two minutes, standing unsupported with one foot in front, standing in one leg, picking up an object from standing position and moving from sit down to standup. Based on the participants' performance for each exercise a grade between 0 and 4 is given. The total score determines the balance condition as follows: a score below 20 indicates poor balance, a score between 21 and 40 indicates fair balance and a score over 40 is considered good. The average BBS score was 49.8 (SD $\pm$ 0.9) which indicates a good baseline balance for the study sample.

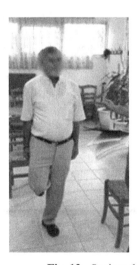
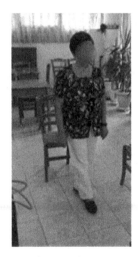

Fig. 12. Seniors during BBS exercises.

The 30SST is a simple exercise to assess the muscle strength of the participants. The senior is asked to sit in a chair and stand up as many times as possible in 30 s without any help. Table 3 provides the 30SST scores per participant for the baseline stage. The average score was 13 (SD $\pm$ 1.7). The overall outcome of the baseline physical condition assessment was that all participants had relatively high scores and therefore there was no high risk of falling during the game.

Table 3. Statistics of BBS and 30SST [23].

Metric	Pre	Post	Diff	p-value
BBS	49.8 ($\pm$0.9)	50.3 ($\pm$0.8)	0.5	0.007
30SST	13 ($\pm$1.7)	13.4 ($\pm$1.2)	0.4	0.05

6.3 Exergaming

During this stage the seniors played the game starting with the easy level and continued to the next one up to the advanced level (Fig. 13). While playing various parameters were recorded like the playing time, the collected points and whether the participant completed the level or stopped and quit. In the initial sessions, while all the participants completed the first and second level, many of them had to stop prematurely the advanced level due to tiredness. After some sessions however they were able to complete all game levels. It is worth mentioning that during this stage there were requests by more seniors of the Elderly Center to play the game. They had the opportunity to play sometimes the game, but their statistics were not recorded because they didn't participate in the study from the beginning.

6.4 Post-exergame Physical Condition Assessment

After the end of the five weeks period the participants repeated the two balance tests to evaluate the effect of exergaming in their performance. Table 3 summarize the results by comparing the baseline and post exergaming scores. The average BBS score after exergaming was improved to 50.3 (SD $\pm$ 0.8) (50% of the participants experienced an improvement in their balance) while the average 30SST score was slightly improved to 13.4 (SD $\pm$ 1.2). Given the good scores from the baseline stage and the limited timeframe of the study the overall balance improvements attained were considered positive.

6.5 Results

The quantitative and qualitative data collected during the study were analyzed to identify the impact of the proposed exergame.

Statistical analysis using Wilcoxon signed-ranks test (due to non-normality of the data) for paired samples and a level of significance (a = 0.05) was applied to compare the BBS and 30SST scores between pre and post exergaming. The results shown in Table 3 indicate that the BBS score improvement between the pre and post exergaming periods is statistically significant ($p < 0.05$), whereas the 30SST score improvement is

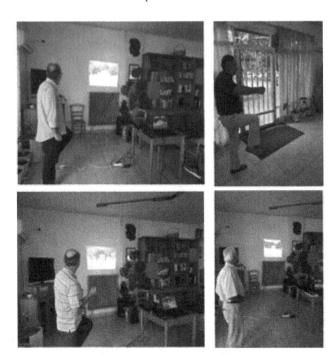

Fig. 13. Seniors playing the game [23].

statistically marginally significant (p = 0.05). The walking and leaning motions included in the exergame design could explain the improvements as these movements contribute in maintaining both motor and balance function.

The performance statistics exported by the system indicated an improvement on the game completion time per level throughout the timeframe of the study. In particular, for the easy level the average completion time for all participants was reduced from 358 to 254 s (29.1%), for the normal level from 540 to 485 s (10.2%) and for the advanced level from 1000 to 917 s (8.3%). Figure 14 illustrates the progress of the average game completion time throughout the study for the three game levels.

Another indicator of participant's interest towards the game is given in Fig. 15 which shows the number of the baskets the players delivered in the advanced level. In the first two weeks due to physical tiredness the average baskets delivered was less than the threshold to complete the level. However, from week 3 until the end of the study all the participants were able to complete the advanced level.

6.6 Usability Assessment

In order to determine the system's usability, short duration interviews and meetings were conducted with both seniors and medical experts in order to assess whether the system had a positive impact and to identify the future features that need to be implemented. The interview with the seniors showed that 100% of the participants found the exergame to be enjoyable, 80% thought that the movements were not complicated but easy to

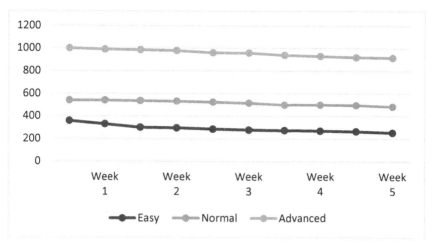

Fig. 14. Average game completion time.

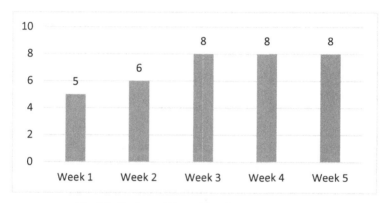

Fig. 15. Baskets delivered in advanced level [23].

remember and 90% of them expressed their expectation to use the exergame after the study.

Positive comments were provided for the game theme and the extensionality of the 3D textures as well as the seamless navigation of the game through the player avatar. Positive comments also provided that their confidence on the technology increased due to their experience with the game tool. The interview with the expert gave the feedback that the use of the game not only helped the seniors to improve their physical state but contributed to the improvement of their psychological and emotional state as they were happy when playing the game and throughout the duration of the study there was a positive feeling and anticipation towards the planned activities.

Besides the semi-structured interviews, users were asked to fill out a questionnaire in order to better investigate and evaluate the degree of which the users were satisfied by the system. The questionnaire was based on the constructs of the Unified Theory of Acceptance and Use of Technology (UTAUT) model [25] as summarized in Table 4. For each of the construct two questions were drafted (see Table 5) with rated response from 1 to 5 with 1 being strongly disagree and 5 being strongly agree.

Table 4. UTAUT constructs used in the study.

Construct	Description
Performance Expectancy (PE)	The degree to which the individuals believe that the use of the technologies will result in performance gains
Effort Expectancy (EE)	The ease of use of the technologies
Social Influence (SI)	The extent to which the individuals believe that others should use the technologies
Facilitating Conditions (FC)	The perceived extent to which the organizational and technical infrastructure required for the support of the technologies exist
Behavioral Intention (BI)	The degree to which the individuals have the intention to use the technology in the future

Table 5. Question items for each category.

Construct	Item Code	Item
Performance Expectancy (PE)	PE1	The system would improve seniors physical condition
	PE2	The system would reduce fall risk
Effort Expectancy (EE)	EE1	The system is easy to use
	EE2	I would need the support of an expert to use this system
Social Influence (SI)	SI1	I think most people will learn to use this system quickly
	SI2	I think most people will enjoy playing this game
Facilitating Conditions (FC)	FC1	I have the necessary resources to use this system
	FC2	I have the necessary knowledge to use this system
Behavioral Intention (BI)	BI1	I intend to use this system in the near future
	BI2	I felt very confident using the system

After collecting the responses to the questionnaire from the seniors we have calculated the Cronbach's Alpha score for each of the categories in order to determine the reliability degree. Table 6 shows the results for each of the model's construct, which is higher than 0.70 which makes the questionnaire that was formed valid and reliable [26].

Table 6. Cronbach's Alpha of the measurement constructs and items.

Category	Cronbach's Alpha	Number of Items
Performance Expectancy (PE)	.802	2
Effort Expectancy (EE)	.787	2
Social Influence (SI)	.797	2
Facilitating Conditions (FC)	.756	2
Behavioral Intention (BI)	.757	2

Descriptive statistics analysis (Table 7) reveals that for the performance expectancy the majority (41.6%) strongly agrees that the system would help seniors improve their physical condition. As for reducing the risk of falling, seniors simply agree that the system could help towards this goal.

Table 7. Descriptive statistics analysis of the measurement constructs and items.

Category	1	2	3	4	5
PE1	0%	0%	16.6%	33.3%	41.6%
PE2	0%	0%	50%	25%	25%
EE1	0%	0%	25%	33.3%	41.6%
EE2	0%	0%	33.3%	50%	16.6%
SI1	0%	0%	33.3%	25%	41.6%
SI2	0%	0%	33.3%	25%	41.6%
FC1	58.3%	16.6%	25%	0%	0%
FC2	50%	33.3%	16.6%	0%	0%
BI1	0%	0%	25%	33.3%	41.6%
BI2	0%	41.6%	25%	25%	8.33%

Furthermore, data from the effort expectancy category show that seniors didn't find the system hard to use but only after they got the appropriate instructions from an expert since they didn't have the knowledge to use the system from the beginning.

As for the social influence, seniors believe that others would benefit from using the game and enjoy such systems which was also reflected during the sessions where some elderly outside the study group showed interest in playing the game. Also, even though the majority of the users do not have the appropriate equipment to use the system, seniors showed a positive attitude towards acquiring the equipment in order to be able to use the system in the near future.

Finally, seniors were asked to fill out the system usability scale (SUS) questionnaire. SUS is a 10-item questionnaire with five response options from strongly disagree to strongly agree [27]. The participant's grades for each item were processed so that the original scores of 0–40 are converted to 0–100. Except from three seniors who rated the exergame tool as acceptable (scores 75–78) all the other scores were above 80. The average SUS score was 84.3 out of 100, suggesting a high user acceptance [28].

7 Discussion

The research conducted and described in this paper argued and provided evidence that exergames for seniors, if properly designed, can be an enjoyable tool for balance training leading to improvements in physical health conditions.

Data analysis from the evaluation study showed that seniors consider such systems can be reliable and used as an alternative mean for improving their physical condition through daily exercise. Also, they believe that the system complexity is low, the exergame is easy to understand on its mechanics and doesn't require much effort to use. Furthermore, users found the required gestures of the game easy to perform and expressed a positive intention to use the designed system in the future and were willing to recommend it to other seniors.

The system achieved a SUS score of 84.3 which means that the interaction mechanisms of the developed system have a good to excellent usability. Also, the post-exergaming physical evaluation of the seniors through BBS and 30SST tests showed a significant improvement according to literature measures compared to the baseline physical assessment. Despite the small sample size, the findings are considered relevant as there are similar levels of improvement to other studies found in the literature [29, 30].

In line with other studies, seniors due to the lack of knowledge for the new technologies often show a hesitation in interacting with it [31, 32]. Despite that, seniors show a positive attitude towards learning to use such systems. Choosing an appropriate game theme as well as providing positive feedback during the game proved to be the main reason for seniors to stay motivated and thus keep progressing in the game.

While other studies focus on developing a two-dimensional world, the development of a three-dimensional open world makes such system more realistic and thus more attractive to use by the elderly. Also, such a world provides motivation to keep playing as it provides the opportunity to explore the game world without being limited in a single place.

From a technological scope, Microsoft Kinect sensor proved to be a reliable device in correctly identifying motions and gestures under any game scenario and providing useful feedback to the user. Thus, low cost commercial sensor devices can be a viable tool for alternative daily exercise. Given the low cost of the sensor device and its portability the tool can be deployed and used in settings ranging from homes to facility centers supporting the elderly.

Limitations of the current study are acknowledged. The limited number of participants and the short evaluation timeframe prevent the justification of more sound results. Achieving substantial balance improvements in elderly requires playing the games over 3 times per week for at least 3 months [29]. In comparison, the duration of this study was 5 weeks with 2 game sessions per week.

8   Conclusion and Future Work

In this work a system that aims to improve seniors' physical condition and balance control through exergaming has been developed using a human centered design approach. A three-dimension world was developed allowing the user to explore various sceneries and not being confined by just completing a level. The evaluation study showed a high usability score and a positive acceptance of the system by the users providing a new and enjoyable way of performing exercises.

Work in progress includes the addition of more game features such as a multiplayer option where players can either work together to complete the game level faster or against each other. Furthermore, the implementation of daily missions (such as "Deliver two baskets under x min") would increase challenges for more demanding users. Figure 16 shows an early development stage of the multiplayer game scenario where the pink colorized object indicates the second player. Our goal is to implement a 3D avatar for each player. In the current scenario the two players work against each other to complete the level.

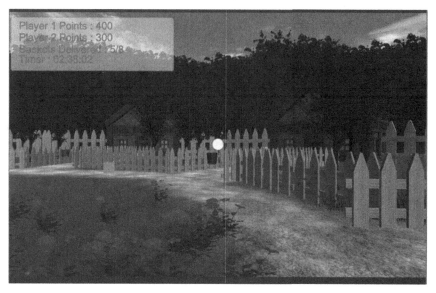

Fig. 16. Early stage of a multiplayer version of the exergames. (Color figure online)

Future plans include the integration of newer technologies like Virtual Reality (VR) in the game mechanics. Furthermore, since VR technology besides requiring an appropriate mask employs also controllers to move the player, designing a scheme that combines other sensors like the Azure Kinect will enable to track the user's gestures without the need of holding extra controllers.

Furthermore, a cognitive assessment dimension is planned to be incorporated with automatic game adaption based on user's characteristics and progression using machine learning techniques which will perform classification of the collected game data. For instance, the new implementation aims to remove the fixed difficulty levels. The aim is to have a system that will adjust its difficulty based on the results from the user's data analysis giving the player extra motivation in playing the game and thus resulting in more training.

Finally, an evaluation study with a larger sample of seniors, including a control group, and for a longer period of time would provide a more sound justification of the present results.

References

1. Lamoth, C.J.C., Caljouw, S.R., Postema, K.: Active video gaming to improve balance in the elderly. Stud. Health Technol. Inform. **167**, 159–164 (2011)
2. Sherrington, C., Tiedemann, A., Fairhall, N., Close, J.C.T., Lord, S.R.: Exercise to prevent falls in older adults: an updated meta-analysis and best practice recommendations. New South Wales Public Health Bull. **22**, 78–83 (2011)
3. Van Diest, M., Lamoth, C.J.C., Stegenga, J., Verkerke, G.J., Postema, K.: Exergaming for balance training of elderly: state of the art and future developments. J. Neuroeng. Rehabil. **10**(1), 101 (2013). https://doi.org/10.1186/1743-0003-10-101
4. Goble, D.J., Cone, B.L., Fling, B.W.: Using the Wii Fit as a tool for balance assessment and neurorehabilitation: the first half decade of "Wii-search". J. Neuroeng. Rehabil. **11**(12), 1–9 (2014). https://doi.org/10.1186/1743-0003-11-12
5. Gerling, K.M., Schulte, F.P., Smeddinck, J., Masuch, M.: Game design for older adults: effects of age-related changes on structural elements of digital games. In: Herrlich, M., Malaka, R., Masuch, M. (eds.) ICEC 2012. LNCS, vol. 7522, pp. 235–242. Springer, Heidelberg (2012). https://doi.org/10.1007/978-3-642-33542-6_20
6. Lange, B., Flynn, S., Rizzo, A.: Initial usability assessment of off-the-shelf video game consoles for clinical game-based motor rehabilitation. Phys. Ther. Rev. **14**(5), 355–363 (2009)
7. Sugarman, H., Weisel-Eichler, A., Burstin, A., Brown, R.: Use of the wii fit system for the treatment of balance problems in the elderly: a feasibility study. In: Virtual Rehabilitation International Conference, pp. 111–116 (2009)
8. Bateni, H.: Changes in balance in older adults based on use of physical therapy vs the Wii Fit gaming system: a preliminary study. Physiotherapy **98**(3), 211–216 (2012)
9. Weisman, S.: Computer games for the frail elderly. Gerontol. **23**(4), 361–363 (1983)
10. Korn, O., Brach, M., Hauer, K., Unkauf, S.: Exergames for elderly persons: physical exercise software based on motion tracking within the framework of ambient assisted living. In: Serious Games and Virtual Worlds in Education, Professional Development, and Healthcare, pp. 258–268 (2013)
11. Garcia, J.A.: Assessing the validity of in-game stepping performance data from a kinect-based fall prevention exergame. In: 6th IEEE International Conference on Serious Games and Applications for Health (SeGAH) (2018)
12. Mousavi Hondori, H., Khademi, M.: A review on technical and clinical impact of microsoft kinect on physical therapy and rehabilitation. J. Med. Eng. **846514**, 2014 (2014)
13. Fu, A.S., Gao, K.L., Tung, A.K., Tsang, W.W., Kwan, M.M.: Effectiveness of exergaming training in reducing risk and incidence of falls in frail older adults with a history of falls. Arch. Phys. Med. Rehabil. **96**(12), 2096–2102 (2015)
14. Kostaki, C., Goumopoulos, C.: Development and evaluation of an exergaming application for improving seniors' well-being. In Proceedings of the 20th Pan-Hellenic Conference on Informatics, p. 27 (2016)

15. Brox, E., Konstantinidis, S.T., Evertsen, G.: User-centered design of serious games for older adults following 3 years of experience with exergames for seniors: a study design. JMIR Serious Games **5**(1), e2 (2017)
16. Sato, K., Kuroki, K., Saiki, S., Nagatomi, R.: Improving walking, muscle strength, and balance in the elderly with an exergame using kinect: a randomized controlled trial. Games Health J. **4**(3), 161–167 (2015)
17. Stanmore, E., et al.: Reducing falls risk with Kinect based falls prevention exergames: a 12 week twocentre, cluster RCT of community-dwelling older adults living in sheltered housing. J. Frailty Sarcopenia Falls, **3**(1) (2018)
18. Mateo, F., Soria-Olivas, E., Carrasco, J., Bonanad, S., Querol, F., Pérez-Alenda, S.: HemoKinect: a microsoft kinect V2 based exergaming software to supervise physical exercise of patients with hemophilia. Sensors **18**(8), 2439 (2018)
19. Pachoulakis, I., Papadopoulos, N., Analyti, A.: Kinect-based exergames tailored to Parkinson patients. Int. J. Comput. Games Technol. (2018)
20. Wever, R., Van Kuijk, J., Boks, C.: User-centred design for sustainable behaviour. Int. J. Sustain. Eng. **1**(1), 9–20 (2008)
21. Gerling, K., Livingston, I., Nacke, L., Mandryk, R.: Full-body motion-based game interaction for older adults. In: SIGCHI Conference on Human Factors in Computing Systems, pp. 1873–1882 (2012)
22. Tashev, I.: Kinect development kit: a toolkit for gesture-and speech-based human-machine interaction. IEEE Sig. Process. Mag. **30**(5), 129–131 (2013)
23. Chartomatsidis, M., Goumopoulos, C.: A balance training game tool for seniors using microsoft kinect and 3D worlds. In: International Conference on Information and Communication Technologies for Ageing Well and e-Health, pp. 135–145 (2019)
24. Berg, K.O., Wood-Dauphinee, S.L., Williams, J.I., Maki, B.: Measuring balance in the elderly: validation of an instrument. Can. J. Public Health **83**, S7–S11 (1992)
25. Venkatesh, V., Zhang, X.: Unified theory of acceptance and use of technology: US vs. China. J. Glob. Inf. Technol. Manag. **13**(1), 5–27 (2010)
26. Sharma, A.K., Kumar, D.: User acceptance of desktop based computer software using UTAUT model and addition of new moderators. Int. J. Comput. Sci. Eng. Technol. 509–515 (2012)
27. Brooke, J.: SUS-A quick and dirty usability scale. Usabil. Eval. Ind. **189**(194), 4–7 (1996)
28. Bangor, A., Kortum, P.T., Miller, J.T.: An empirical evaluation of the system usability scale. Int. J. Hum.-Comput. Interact. **24**(6), 574–594 (2008)
29. Wüest, S., Borghese, N.A., Pirovano, M., Mainetti, R., van de Langenberg, R., de Bruin, E.D.: Usability and effects of an exergame-based balance training program. Games Health: Res. Dev. Clin. Appl. **3**(2), 106–114 (2014)
30. Agmon, M., Perry, C.K., Phelan, E., Demiris, G., Nguyen, H.Q.: A pilot study of wii fit exergames to improve balance in older adults. J. Geriatr. Phys. Ther. **34**(4), 161–167 (2011)
31. Čaić, M., Rodrigues, V., Holmlid, S., Mahr, D., Odekerken-Schröder, G.: Exergames for healthy ageing: inclusion through design. In Proceedings of the Design4Health, pp. 235–238 (2017)
32. Iversen, S.M.: Play and productivity: the constitution of ageing adults in research on digital games. Games Cult. **11**(1–2), 7–27 (2016)

The Technology-Enhanced Requirements for the Three-Fold Stroke Rehabilitation to Support Independent Living

Awais Ahmad[✉], Karin Ahlin, and Peter Mozelius

Department of Computer and System Science, Mid Sweden University, Östersund, Sweden
{awais.ahmad,karin.ahlin,peter.mozelius}@miun.se

Abstract. Stroke is a common and severe disease that can be found in all regions across the globe, and not only among older adults. Result of a stroke can be death, or a variety of disabilities caused by impairments in different brain functions. This chapter discusses technology enhanced stroke rehabilitation from a three-fold view of cognitive, motoric and speech rehabilitation. The important research question was: What would be the requirements for technology-enhanced stroke rehabilitation in the areas of cognitive, motoric and speech rehabilitation? The study was carried out with a requirement-focused Design Science approach collecting data with semi-structured interviews. Informants were selected in a purposive sampling choosing professionals with valuable knowledge and skills in stroke rehabilitation. The findings in this study have generated useful general requirements for a future implementation and testing of technology enhanced stroke rehabilitation. Within each of the three rehabilitation categories cognitive, motoric and speech, there seems to be potential for successful use of technology enhanced services. This development of rehabilitation services must follow the fundamental principle for all forms of stroke rehabilitation: each patient needs a personalised treatment. However, in all three rehabilitation categories, there is a need to define more specific requirements based on feedback from stroke patients testing the rehabilitation services.

Keywords: e-Health · Stroke rehabilitation · Independent living · Speech rehabilitation · Physio rehabilitation · Cognitive rehabilitation

1 Introduction

Discussed in a previous article (Ahmad et al. 2019), were general requirements for stroke rehabilitation. Here we present a more detailed three-fold view on the topic. Moreover, in the previous article, there were five semi-structured interviews, and here they are extended to twelve. The core theme and aim of this article corresponds closely to those in the previous article, with the addition of a more detailed view, stronger results, and more nuanced findings.

Stroke is one of the most common and severe diseases across the globe resulting in death or a variety of disabilities (Langhorne et al. 2011). Stroke is caused by an

© Springer Nature Switzerland AG 2020
M. Ziefle and L. A. Maciaszek (Eds.): ICT4AWE 2019, CCIS 1219, pp. 142–159, 2020.
https://doi.org/10.1007/978-3-030-52677-1_8

interruption of blood flow to the brain that affects neuronal cells, which leads to severe impairments in brain function (Toussignant et al. 2018). Stroke, in its initial phase, is treated in emergency care and with immediate planning on how and where to rehabilitate the patient. After the emergency treatment, the rehabilitation starts, and it is founded on the details of the patient's condition and their wishes and motivation for a better life (Dimaguila et al. 2018) and society's goals for a better life and health (UN 2019). Because of the injuries, quality of life is severely compromised, and a patient's social interaction decreases since these changes have a long-lasting impact on the patient's personal and professional life. The rehabilitation has to be carried out throughout every day of their life and should not be dependent on variations in the patient's environment. Added to this need for patients' independence are the unsurprising findings that most older adults prefer to age well and live independently, which is also favored policy makers (Peek et al. 2016). Ageing well, or healthy ageing, has been described as a lifelong process of optimising opportunities for improving and preserving health and physical, social and mental wellness to obtain independence and quality of life (Peel et al. 2004). Stroke is one of several acute health conditions that often results in lost independence, so a main objective in any rehabilitation must be to reestablish and facilitate patients' independent living to recapture their quality of life (Gwozdz and Sousa-Poza 2010).

Generally, a stroke patient's disability can be classified into motor, speech and cognitive injuries, where the cognitive part is intertwingled with motor and speech. This paper handles all three categories of disabilities, where cognitive deals with problems handling everyday mental activities, motor deals with problems in using the body, and speech deals with problems with language and communication, reducing drastically a person's ability to speak, listen, read and write (Seniów et al. 2009, Langhorne et al. 2011, Veerbeek et al. 2014, Pollock et al. 2014, Toussignant et al. 2018). Traditional treatments offered by a therapist mainly cover everyday therapy, but it is challenging to provide access to those treatments to all stroke patients because a high amount of human resources and running costs are needed for these intervention types. In the last two decades, Technology Enhanced Systems (TES) have emerged as highly useful for several treatments involving multiple rehabilitation therapies (Ahmad et al. 2019).

Due to brain function impairments, the patient's ability to understand and learn new things is decreased drastically, which makes it difficult for patients to adopt and use TES. Added to the patient's perspective is that of the therapist, aiming to support the patient in developing and maintaining the necessary motivation for his/her therapy. Therefore, the users' requirements need to be considered with these perspectives in mind and a user-centred design approach may be most effective (Pagliari 2007; Glasgow, 2007; Dabbs et al. 2009; Neuhauser et al. 2013). Hence, determining requirements are essential for the successful use of TES. The aim of the study was therefore to investigate requirements for the various areas of technology-enhanced stroke rehabilitation and the addressed research question: What would be the requirements for technology-enhanced stroke rehabilitation in the areas of cognitive, motoric and speech rehabilitation?

Although challenges for stroke rehabilitation are prevalent all over the world, our primary focus was the Mid Sweden region, a sparsely populated part of Sweden. According to "Statistics Sweden" is the population of Mid Sweden Region scattered across the whole region and a large number of people are living outside the cities (SCB, 2016).

Consequently, providing rehabilitation services in the remote areas is even more challenging, and a large number of resources are needed to meet these challenges. Therefore, TES can play a vital role in the region.

1.1 Previous Knowledge of Stroke Rehabilitation and Use of TES

Previous knowledge is here divided into cognitive, motoric, and speech rehabilitation. Each section describes the main features of each rehabilitation and the requirements for TES. For the various rehabilitation orientations is it of importance to start the rehabilitation as soon as possible after the stroke to motivate the patient in its individual rehabilitation plan. By using TES could the patient's motivation increase as well as the efficiency for the therapist, especially in sparsely populated areas such as Mid Sweden.

1.2 Cognitive Rehabilitation

The cognitive status of a patient plays a vital role in the process of overall rehabilitation after a stroke, therefore, it is important to examine the condition of a patient's cognition before any intervention (Skidmore et al. 2010, Heruti et al. 2002). Many stroke rehabilitation exercises need cognitive abilities for learning, memorizing and practicing different tasks and any kind of cognitive deficiency can make it difficult to perform these tasks and exercises (Heruti et al. 2002). Therefore, the cognitive skills of patients determine the overall strategy of rehabilitation following a stroke.

The majority of stroke survivors are reported to have cognitive impairments that can severely impact patients' daily life activities (Palmcrantz et al. 2017, Gamito et al. 2017), and a large number of patients need long-term cognitive rehabilitation (Cogollor et al. 2018). After a stroke, even mild cognitive impairments can affect patients' independent living, quality of life and occupational effectiveness (Jokinen et al. 2015). Due to the brain damage, cognitive impairments can cause attention deficits, memory loss, perceptual disorders, and spatial neglect, where some types of training can improve the attention and alertness time for patients with attention deficiencies (Langhorne et al. 2011, Jokinen et al. 2015). Several types of therapies can be suggested for effecting cognitive improvements; their selection, depends on each patient's impairments.

Occupational therapy is one of the traditional and important interventions for cognitive rehabilitation where a patient performs some selected tasks guided by an occupational therapist's visual and verbal cues (Pastorino et al. 2014). Usually, traditional cognitive training for performing these daily routine tasks consists of pen-and-paper exercises (Gamito et al. 2017). Several studies highlight that occupational therapy can improve cognition and daily life activities (Pastorino et al. 2014, Langhorne et al. 2011). Occupational therapy based training and interventions within a few weeks after stroke have the most effective outcome and play an effective role in future rehabilitation, therefore, some kind of therapy should be started as soon as possible following stroke (Ahmad et al. 2019, Pastorino et al. 2014). Even a small improvement in the cognitive state during the first weeks after stroke can make a huge impact on a patient's overall health and future rehabilitation process (Vourvopoulos et al. 2013). However, traditional rehabilitation, operated by therapists, requires a lot of human resources and come with high operational costs (Zhang et al. 2016). In this context, cognitive therapies and exercises based on TES can be helpful to reduce human intervention and operational costs.

A number of research studies suggest that TES have a progressively important role in cognitive rehabilitation following stroke (Gamito et al. 2017, Ahmad et al. 2019, Vourvopoulos et al. 2013). For example, interactive eHealth applications based on virtual reality and game-based learning can improve the patient's memory and attention deficiencies (Vourvopoulos et al. 2013, Gamito et al. 2017). Traditional paper and pencil exercises to restore cognition can be replaced by interactive gaming applications (Gamito et al. 2017). Serious game application based on virtual reality can be developed and effectively used for different daily routine activities (Gamito et al. 2017, Vourvopoulos et al. 2013). A study highlighted that TES helped patients to perform error free daily tasks, for example, making tea became easy for them with the help of an interactive web application (Pastorino et al. 2014). In order to support a patient-centric treatment approach, such applications can be customized according to the patients' needs and cognitive state (Vourvopoulos et al. 2013). Since these applications can be operated and monitored from a distance via internet as well, the patients can use them in their home environment and that support the idea of independent living (Gamito et al. 2017).

1.3 Motoric Rehabilitation

Almost all stroke patients suffer from some kind of motoric impairment, and to start the motoric rehabilitation early is a crucial key activity for most stroke survivors (Langhorne et al. 2009).

The rehabilitation of motor functions, and especially the movement of upper limbs is crucial in the effort for patients to live independently (Stinear and Byblow 2014). Several research studies highlight the importance of an early rehabilitation start, and also the need for an individually adapted long-term plan (Palmcrantz et al. 2017, Ahmad et al. 2019). The common recommendations for motoric rehabilitation are physiotherapy and controlled exercises (Veerbeek et al. 2014), and to obtain good results the physical training should be intense, customised, task-oriented and in high dosage (Palmcrantz et al. 2017). This makes the role of occupational therapists and physiotherapists very important to obtain a well-planned and individually adapted motor recovery (Langhorne et al. 2009).

Today, motoric stroke rehabilitation could be carried out in a mix of traditional rehabilitation, technology enhanced rehabilitation (Parker and Mawson 2017), robot aided rehabilitation (Orihuela-Espina et al. 2016) or game-based rehabilitation (Choi et al. 2016). This study had a focus on how technology enhanced and game-based exercises might complement traditional rehabilitation. In the 21st century, rapid technological development has enabled new ICT technology enhanced solutions for physical rehabilitation (Nicolau et al. 2013). For motoric stroke rehabilitation a wide variety of TES solutions has been developed and evaluated. Some trends have been virtual reality applications with specialised hardware devices (Boian et al. 2002; Wade and Winstein 2011), robot assisted rehabilitation (Wade and Winstein 2011; Orihuela-Espina et al. 2016) and various game-based TES approaches (Alankus et al. 2010; Choi et al. 2016).

Since effective stroke rehabilitation must be intensive and repetitive, patient motivation and engagement is a crucial factor. Digital games have been recognised for their motivational effect, and for motoric stroke rehabilitation an engaging and serious game can be more important than expensive high-end graphics. (Burke et al. 2009) During the last decades, there has been a fast and heterogeneous development of the type of digital games that Juul (2010) calls 'casual games'. His main categories of casual games are: 1) games with mimetic interfaces, and 2) online downloadable casual games. Games with mimetic interfaces often involve physical activities where players mimic an activity that is displayed on the screen. Examples of games with mimetic interfaces with are tennis and bowling on a Wii platform, or an imitation of guitar playing in Guitar Hero. These games are classified as casual since all presumptive players can look at the game and quickly understand the basic game idea. These are interesting aspects for stroke patients since motoric rehabilitation should be based on physical activities, and stroke patients often have reduced cognitive abilities making more complex gameplay hard to learn.

1.4 Speech Rehabilitation

After a stroke, most speech and language impairments are recovered during the first few weeks, but recovery might take several years; several studies highlight that speech and language therapy are effective interventions to enhance the recovery process (Gerstenecker and Lazar 2019). Difficulties related to speech are classified in the conditions of aphasia, dysarthria, and verbal apraxia.

Aphasia is one of the typical stroke impairments where a patient's cognitive performance is decreased, referring to the struggle with understanding what a word means, finding the right word to use, and using grammar correctly (Toussignant et al. 2018). This cognitive performance refers to the abilities to speak, read and write to various extents. Almost one-third of patients tend to have aphasia after a stroke (Brady et al. 2016). Dysarthria refers to impairment in the muscles used to speak and can affect pronunciation or phonation. Verbal apraxia refers to difficulties in planning what and how to say something. Stroke patients can suffer from all impairments in varying degrees as well as suffering from only one of them.

Several studies confirmed that the quality of life of people with chronic speech impairments is severely affected because of their emotional suffering, social limitations, and communication disorders (Hilari et al. 2003; Ross and Wertz 2003; Öra et al. 2018). The stroke patients can no longer express their emotions, opinions, thoughts, personality and knowledge, and that lack of expression leads to deep frustration (Johansson et al. 2012). Another impact of speech inability is the feeling of uncertainty and fear. The patients become uncertain about what is said and what is understood, leading to doubts about what was planned in the past and continuous fear of future unpleasant situations. Consequently, this devastating disability impacts the people living around the patient, such as relatives and friends (Öra et al. 2018). Therefore, speech therapy is important for stroke patients and some evidence has shown that highly intensive, highly dosed, and long-term therapies have better results than low intensity, low dosed and short-term therapy (Öra et al. 2018).

TES is one answer to address the need for intensive, highly dosed, and long-term speech therapy. The functional requirements for a TES related to speech rehabilitation should be personalised based on the patient's condition and intention (Simic et al. 2016; Kesav et al. 2017). Simic et al. (2016) describe the need for user-centred design based on the patient's various conditions, emphasising that most TES for speech training assumes that stroke patients do have some base level of language left. Patient's intention refers to the wish for rehabilitation, where stroke patients' motivation for recovery varies. Therefore, the TES should be joyful to use, especially since stroke patients mainly suffer from fatigue and therefore need extra motivation to train (Rybarczyk and Fonseca 2011). The motivation could be based on follow up situations where training results in various gratifications. As such, functionality for follow-ups is of interest and game-based interventions, both from the patient's and the speech therapist's perspective (Rybarczyk and Fonseca 2011; Simic et al. 2016).

Rybarczyk and Fonseca (2011) state that the TES should be based on therapeutic material and be designed according to different levels of language complexity. One part of required functionality is object identification; primarily including simple order comprehension, followed by complex order comprehension (Rybarczyk and Fonseca 2011). The simple order comprehension is based on the construction of a sentence, including name-verb-direct complement. One such example is: "Put the apple behind the folder." Added to the compound sentence is a coordinate or a subordinate sentence, e.g., "Put the apple behind the folder and the orange to the left of the folder. next to the pear." Rybarczyk et al. (2013) add functionality to the order comprehension, where they emphasise that the TES should include the ability to train writing exercises and text, word selections, and specific questions. The order for the writing exercises, or any exercise, should be natural to change for the speech therapist, offering various ways for developing the training. Besides the requirements as mentioned earlier, is it discussed that the training must be based on the patient's mother tongue; mainly related to the fact that several training programs only are available in, e.g. English (Rybarczyk et al. 2013; Kesav et al. 2017).

There are several described non-functional requirements, such as the user control interface where the stroke patient often has motor disabilities and the possibility to use a tablet for training (Mallet et al. 2019). There are some examples of support for motor disabilities, such as simplified graphical layout (Rybarczyk and Fonseca 2011). The graphical layout supporting stroke patients should be as easy as possible to use relating to the patient's condition and include oral and written instructions or possibilities for assistance from another person. One possible solution for assistance is that of a joystick, where the stroke patient can adjust the control sensitivity (Rybarczyk et al. 2013). The wish for a tablet as a device is based on its easiness to use for more than one person, where relatives could be of importance for the stroke patient while using the tablet. Another aspect of the tablet is during communication, where this smaller device offers significant support. One such situation for communication is the description or discussion between two persons where pointing at a picture on a tablet is natural.

2   Method

This study was conducted with a Design Science approach that was inspired by the five-step process described by Johannesson and Perjons (2014). Design Science could be defined as a thorough process where an identified problem should be addressed by the design and implementation of an artefact to make research contributions (Hevner

et al. 2004, Peffers et al. 2007, Johannesson and Perjons 2014). In this study, the first
two phases of the selected process are used. The process is described below in Figure 1.
The first step was to identify and formulate a problem and testbed design requirements
were defined in the second step.

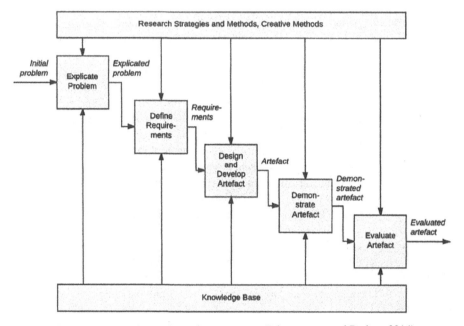

Fig. 1. Phases in the Design science process (Johannesson and Perjons 2014).

2.1 Data Collection

The most common approach to collect data for determining the requirements is often
some kind of interviews. By selecting and then interviewing different stockholders
according to their expertise and background may lead us to the requirements specification. Although interviews can be effective but if they are too structured, informant's
creativity and freedom of expression may be compromised. Therefore, unstructured or
semi-structured interviews are considered as a best practice to encourage informant's
creativeness. Moreover, the selection of informants with right competence and attitude
is also important in the process of requirement specification (Johannesson and Perjons
2014).

In this study, semi-structured interviews combined with a literature study were used
to gather the data for requirements specification. All the interviews were conducted by
following a basic question schedule that was further customized for different informants
according to their skills and professional background. The basic themes for the interview
question included the informants' current knowledge, basic work routines and responsi-
bilities in stroke rehabilitation, their understanding and perceived usefulness of e-health

services, their expectations from ICT and the financial aspects of using ICT. Keywords such as stroke rehabilitation, e-health, independent living, speech rehabilitation, physio rehabilitation, and cognitive rehabilitation were used for conducting a literature review. Some notes were also written during the interviews that not only complemented the audio recordings but also used in the data analysis process.

A purposive sampling approach was adopted for the informants' selection where all the informants have exceptional knowledge and skills in stroke rehabilitation. Purposive sampling refers to a selection technique where researchers choose interviewees based on their own judgment. The design science idea of expert opinions refers that the informants should be selected carefully according to their knowledge and expertise in the given field of research (Wieringa 2014). Data were collected in semi-structured interviews with ten informants which roles in stroke rehabilitation are described below in Table 1.

Table 1. Informants and their years of experience of Stroke rehabilitation.

Informant	Professional role	Years of experience
Informant 1	Speech therapist #1	25
Informant 2	The region's medically responsible doctor	25
Informant 3	Occupational therapist	5
Informant 4	Physiotherapist #1	8
Informant 5	Physiotherapist #2	3
Informant 6	Chairman of the local stroke patient organisation	3
Informant 7	Speech therapist #2	4
Informant 8	CEO of a small company working with game-based stroke rehabilitation	25
Informant 9	Hardware and software specialist at a big multinational company	9
Informant 10	Head of Stroke Team	15

Informants 3, 4, 5, and 10 are part of the mobile stroke rehabilitation team which is located at the region's hospital. This mobile team consists of a manager and four co-workers with different kind of competencies in stroke rehabilitation. The team responsible for the post-clinical rehabilitation after patients have been relocated to their homes. However, this service can be offered to patients living within the 70 km area from the main region's hospital. Informant 3,4,5 and 7 have been interviewed twice to gather some more detailed information and to ask some further questions that raised after the initial interviews.

2.2 Data Analysis

A deductive thematic analysis approach was adopted to discover the themes and patterns that were useful to establish the requirements for technology-enhanced stroke rehabilitation in the areas of speech, motor, and cognitive rehabilitation. Initially, each researcher analysed the interview material individually and then some combined discussions on the individual analysis were conducted to conclude the important themes and findings. The individual analysis was conducted by the steps: meaning units, condensation, code, category, and themes. (Erlingsson and Brysiewicz, 2017, Bengtsson, 2016, Elo and Kyngäs 2008). The most important findings from the analyses that are relevant to the research question are presented in the findings section.

2.3 Ethical Considerations

One part of being a researcher is to consider ethics, namely how to conscientiously deal with people taking part in your research and the consequences of the research you are doing (Helgesson 2015). Discussed in research ethics, as well as in ordinary life, is morality, with arguments about the meanings of good, bad, right or wrong. Research ethics is categorised as professional ethics, which the Swedish Research Council (CODEX 2016) describes in three general subsets. They are: (1) conducting good work, (2) follow national and local rules, and (3) follow professional codes of ethics. The third subset includes parts such as the researcher should work in close collaboration with user groups to satisfy them, show the user groups respect, focus on healthy work environments, and protect the individuals from harm (Dahlbom and Mathiassen, 2017). Here, it has been done in various steps, where one is to the users' voices by interviewing them and rephrasing their well-informed voices to shared and accessible knowledge. Another way, which should be viewed as directed towards the overall aim of this study, is that of creating a healthy work environment for the stroke patients and the therapists by focusing on their specific requirements for TES.

The primary empirical material in this thesis is collected through interviews. Therefore, it is of interest to discuss the ethics for interviews. Kvale and Brinkmann (2014) discuss them in various steps. One is the informed consent, and their secured confidentiality is by not using either the organisations' or participants' real names. At the introduction of interviews, the researcher(s) have informed the respondent of their voluntary participation in the interview, their right to not answer a particular question, and the right to withdraw from the interview at any time. All interviews were recorded, stored where a password is required, and transcribed verbatim by the researchers.

The transcription, which Kvale and Brinkmann (2014) propose to secure the respondent's confidentiality and transcriptions loyal to their answers. The time-consuming transcription is made verbatim to give the real answers from the respondents. Transcribing verbatim is usually not the problem; the construction of sentences is more laborious. One of the last steps for interview ethics is the analysis. Kvale and Brinkmann (2014) discuss how much the researcher can put into the respondents' answers. Here, this is a question to be answered on a general level – how do we interpret our material and how can we generalise in interpretative research. Turning focus to the interview material, it has been shared with and discussed among all researchers as well as researchers in the domain of e-health, mainly at various conferences.

3 Findings

Described below are findings from the informants divided into the three rehabilitation paths. All informants highlight the importance of TES being built on the patient's need and that there is a difference in how the stroke patient can use a TES in comparison to a healthy person, mainly due to the stroke but also related to the TES' interface and functionality. One example is the stroke patient's brain fatigue, where it should be easy to resume any rehabilitation program in a TES.

3.1 Cognitive Rehabilitation

Most of the informants highlighted the importance of early diagnosis of patient's cognitive abilities and current state of brain functions after stroke where patient's current mental and physical condition should be considered while designing TES for stroke survivors (Informant 1–6, 7 and 9). Generally, a patient's ability to understand, express and perform can be determined by on his cognitive state. As highlighted by informant 1, patient's ability to perform different tasks and exercises heavily depends on the degree of brain damage and cognitive state after stroke, therefore, patient's cognitive skills should be examined first and then an individual exercise plan should be adopted based on that examination (Informant 1, 2). For example, patients with a minor cognitive disability can use text-based and complex technology-enhanced applications independently; on the other hand, patients with severe brain damage are suggested to use simple and image-based technology-enhanced application where they might need extra guidance and help from a therapist (Informant 1).

Due to impaired cognition and memory loss, the ability to recognize different things can be affected, therefore, unfamiliar and complex graphical user interfaces can be challenging for the patients (Informant 3, 6, and 7). Informant 6 and 3 mentioned that the stroke patients have to relearn many things due to memory loss and in this situation, learning and navigating new and complex interfaces can be very difficult for them. Therefore, TES should be easy to operate and interactive. As suggested by informant 7, simple and interactive web or mobile applications should be used where daily routine tasks can be practiced such as going to a departmental store or making a cup of coffee.

The informants from computer science and technology background suggested that TES should be and can be adopted according to the different patients' needs (Informant 8, 9). Informant 9 discussed the possibilities of multiplatform applications that can be installed and used on a different kind of hardware and software such as mobiles, tablets, and desktop computers so that a device can be suggested according to the current availability of ICT and patient's medical condition. Technologies such as motion sensors or deep learning cameras connected to a TV or LED screen can be used in the home environment to play interactive games (Informant 8, 9) and those interactive games can be used to relearn different daily life activities and to perform other different kind rehabilitation exercises. Especially, older adults can be great beneficiaries of this kind of technologies.

Different kinds of web or mobile applications can help older people to improve their cognition and daily life actives but the use of these applications depends upon their current health condition and ease of use of the application (informant 1). The older adults seem to have even more cognitive issues, that makes it difficult for them to use TES (informant 1–3). Some older adults are actually against the use of TES in health interventions and they do not even want to try eHealth applications (informant 2). The reason could be lack of knowledge and perceived benefit of using those applications (informant 1). Therefore they need more education, training, and motivation than the younger population (informant 1).

3.2 Motoric Rehabilitation

All interviewees stressed the importance of that TES requirements must always have an individual adaptation to each actual stroke patient where the degree of damage after stroke, age, overall health condition and previous experiences of TES play an important role to determine the requirements for a patient (Informant 1–10). Informant 1 mentioned that the use of TES applications depends on to what degree a patient's brain is affected by stroke. This is of great importance for the motoric rehabilitation, but must also be considered for speech rehabilitation and cognitive rehabilitation.

More specific for the motoric rehabilitation stroke patients' reduced upper limb movements could need software navigation by eye-tracking technology (Informant 2). Another alternative suggested by Informant 9 is voice recognition technology for patients with reduced mobility, and that the patient just can tell the desktop computer to start the actual rehabilitation application, without any physical input (Informant 9). For some patients with reduced upper limb functionality sensor technology might also be helpful for navigation in TES applications (Informant 8, 9), with the idea of patients interacting with a device by the use of hand movements (Informant 9). There are also several requirements from the caregiver perspective. One is the possibility to provide individualised assignments, with a focus on the desired development for every specific patient (Informant 2, 5, 6, and 7). Other caregiver requirements are that the assignments need to be based on caregivers' professional skills, and that all exercises should be safe to conduct. Informant 7 described the idea of how a physiotherapist can use a combination of video and images in motoric exercises to illustrate the optimum angle for a specific movements.

TES services should both be interesting and joyful to use (Informant 1, 2). The design of TES services must consider patients with brain and physical dysfunctions should be able to use these services (Informant 2). Furthermore, Informant 2 strongly emphasised the importance of designing or joyfulness and usability, and that patients can experience senses of happiness while doing useful TES exercises. with the help of TES and should feel the perceived benefits of those exercises (Informant 2). The Informants with more technical backgrounds suggested TES services with motion sensors or deep cameras combined with screens with built-in software in where a patient can play interactive games in their home environments (Informant 8, 9). Informant 5 and Informant 6 also found the idea of using games in the motoric rehabilitation interesting, and asked for dancing games and virtual golfing.

As Informant 1 pointed out, there are no existing games that can fit all stroke patients. There are huge variations in stroke patients' cognitive abilities, physical abilities as well as in their digital literacy. As an example, the full field of view could be blurred which would make some types of gaming problematic. Sophisticated and complex graphical user interfaces might also be troublesome to learn and to use for post-stroke patients. Informant 6 highlighted that stroke patients also often have to relearn, and with various daily skills to relearn, it might be hard to also learn how to use new and unknown digital interfaces (Informant 3, Informant 6). Complex games with complicated game-play should be avoided and the same goes for long gaming sessions for a target group with limited energy. The idea of using well-designed and user-friendly casual games looks promising both for exergames such as virtual table-tennis on large screens, and for mobile games to play at anytime and anywhere. Finally, the requirements mentioned above for game-based exercises should of course be considered for all other types of TES services for stroke rehabilitation.

3.3 Speech Rehabilitation

After a stroke is a person's ability to understand, express, and communicate limited. Therefore, should medically educated professionals be involved in the development of TES for speech rehabilitation to cover the needs and limitations of stroke patients (Informant 7). The overall needs are described as read, write, understand language and speech related to words, sentences, and structure. Today, non-medical professionals develop most of the TES for speech rehabilitation, which can severely affect the usability of the TES (Informant 7). One primary function is that the TES should have the ability to be altered and adjusted accordingly to the patient's medical condition (informant 1, 2, 7). They emphasised that the TES should be easy to use, and patients should feel a sense of joyfulness by using TES (Informant 1, 2).

The requirements for stroke patients with speech problems were divided into two main categories (Informant 1, 7). That is, applications may support communication or training, where the latter includes training of words or meaning structure. The communication problems can be reduced in various ways; for example, by using images or other alternative ways of communication. As in all stroke rehabilitation, the needs vary greatly, resulting in considerable requirement variation for the TES. The lack of TES for easy communication was evident since the demonstrated ones were adjusted for children in elementary school. Informant 7 described that most of the currently available TES are developed for school-going children, and the speech therapists used them after making adjustments. The content was not adjusted for situations in adult lives; for example, communication to describe daily routine work with various degrees of difficulty was missing. The daily routines, such as having a cup of coffee or going to the grocery store, are missing and the adjustment to various degrees of difficulty.

For training, Informant 1 and 7 expressed the following variations on speech problems for the stroke patient: dysphagia (problems with swallowing), aphasia (see earlier description), and dysarthria (reduced mobility in the muscles used in speech). The initial speech problems are mainly related to dysphagia since the patient does not recognise how to swallow. Informant 7 shows a TES supporting training to swallow, which has English narration. While using this TES, Informant 7 turns off the sound and talks to the patient in Swedish. Patients with severe aphasia may suffer from complete loss of speech function; therefore, pictures and video-clips based applications can be helpful (Informant 1, 7). For less damaged patients, voice recording and replaying functions in

TES are recommended that can improve speech function and pronunciation. An interesting finding is that several informants emphasise the importance of considering the patient's vision. Many TES have been developed for persons with a full field of view. For many stroke patients, the full field of view is blurred, creating problems while using many TES. For stroke patients with dysphagia, unknown and complex graphical user interfaces can also be troublesome to learn and accept since they have problems with muscles. For all stroke patients is that they have to relearn, and in a situation where many things should be relearnt, it can be hard also to learn how to navigate in new user interfaces (Informant 3, Informant 6). One solution to this could be to use navigation with, e.g. their eyes.

The requirements from the speech therapist's side were several where the fundamental was proper education and training to use the TES (Informant 1–5, 7). The speech therapist needs to understand all functionality in the TES and how to adjust it to the need for each patient. Informant 7 gives an example by declaring the need on how to mix interactive pictures and video-clips for training instructions. The speech therapists also needed training on more advanced technology for communication, such as Skype or Zoom (Informant 2, 7, and 10). The speech therapist had to make instructions for the stroke patients on how to use those communication tools, such as how to show a video clip at the same time as instructing the stroke patient or relative. The instructions should be easy enough to follow for the stroke patients with their disabilities and perhaps limited knowledge on how to use TES. Importance of proper education and training is even more vital for stroke patients, who often are older adults. Older adults with limited previous e-technology knowledge/experience tend to have more difficulties to use TES than the younger people who have better knowledge/experience of these kinds of technologies (Informant 1–5, 7). Not specifically related to the TES, but still of importance, was the speech therapist's understanding of the stroke patient's privacy and how to access their private information (Informant 1–5, 7).

Added to the work assignments for the speech therapist, was the lack of speech therapists working at the centre for accessibility aid. At prescribing a tablet or a software for speech rehabilitation, there were rarely correctly adjusted for the stroke patient. Therefore, the prescribing speech therapist needs to configure both of them by themselves, which is time-consuming. Discussed by Informant 1, 3, and 6 was also the closely related concept of Bring Your Own Device (BYOD). They referred to it as the users are willing and interested in using their own devices, mainly mobile phones and tablets. The requirements for mobile phones varied; informant 1 relied on applications for ordinary mobile phones, while informant 4 used applications requiring a smartphone with support for email and web login.

4 Discussion

The overall aim of this research was to determine the requirements to use TES for cognitive, motoric and speech rehabilitation following a stroke. To our knowledge, this is the first study to specify the TES requirements for three-fold stroke rehabilitation where a Requirement-Focused Design Science approach was adopted and professionals from both medical and technical backgrounds were interviewed. However, some studies highlighted the importance of user-centered design for interactive eHealth technologies (Dabbs et al. 2009, Simic et al. 2016) and that was completely endorsed by all the informants in this research as well (Informant 1–10).

Although stroke impairments and rehabilitation are classified into three different categories and there are different kinds of therapists for different types of impairments, most of the basic notified requirements to use TES were common. That was an interesting finding since most of the interviews were conducted separately with the informants of different kinds of professional backgrounds. However, some specific requirements are also noted based on the degree of damage after stroke.

The use of TES for all three stroke rehabilitation categories seems to have some obvious benefits. Some recent research studies established that eHealth technologies such as virtual reality (Gamito et al. 2017), serious game-based learning (Choi et al. 2016), telerehabilitation (Tousignant et al. 2018, Øra et al. 2018) and web-based therapy from distance (Simic et al. 2016) can be useful for different kind of interventions following stroke. However, patient's physical and mental condition need to be considered while designing those TES where patent's current medical condition determines his ability to use different kind of treatments (Pollock et al. 2014). As highlighted by all the informants from a medical background, the requirements for TES are not the same for all the stroke survivors. Different factors such as a patient's cognitive, motoric and speech condition after stroke, age, overall physical and mental condition, professional and social life, and previous experience and skills to use TES plays a vital role for requirement speciation (Informants 1–5,7,10). Furthermore, the informants from a technical background not only agreed upon the above statement, but they also suggest different kinds of technologies for different types of patients (Informants 8, 9). As proposed by the CEO of an organization working with game-based stroke rehabilitation, interactive games built on motion sensor technologies can be used in a home environment for motoric therapies (Informants 8). Eye-tracking technology can, of course, help seriously infected patients with serious speech and motor impairments (informant 7, 9).

Age factor should also be considered while designing TES for stroke rehabilitation. Different age groups can have a different kind of needs and exceptions from technology. For example, elderly population find it more challenging to use TES than the younger population (Ahmad and Mozelius). Due to age-related impairments and potential of social isolation, the process of rehabilitation can be more difficult for the elderly population and they tend to suffer from even more cognitive issues such as memory loss (informant 1, 2). Therefore, easy to use, interactive and well-guided eHealth systems are even more important for older adults. Another example of the compromised age factor is observed during an interview at a rehabilitation center in the Mid Sweden region where speech therapists are using some eHealth applications for speech rehabilitation that are basically developed for school children. The tasks and exercises in those applications can be joyful and stimulating for children but might be uninteresting for adults. The adult people found these applications boring and sometimes irrelevant, therefore, TES should be tailor-made and designed for the respective users (informant 7).

What several informants mentioned was the large variation in both stroke patients' rehabilitation needs, and in their digital skills. Considering this, a fundamental idea must be to strive for a smorgasbord with a rich variation of both analogue and TES services. For some patients, it would be both joyful and useful to play virtual golf, for others the best choice might be traditional speech exercises. In the rapid technological development it is tempting to invest in sophisticated devices with motion detection and high-end audio, but stroke patients' limited motoric and cognitive abilities might reduce the benefits of interacting with complex TES environments. Furthermore, the hardware and the software requirements should not only involve patients' requirements, but also consider caregivers and patients' relatives. Several research studies have pointed out the importance of informing and involving stroke patients' relatives (Lomer and McLellan 1987; Almborg et al. 2009; Arntzen and Hamran 2016).

Stroke rehabilitation must always be individually adapted and the trendy concept of Bring Your Own Device (BYOD) seems promising and worth testing in this context. The basic idea in BYOD is learners, or patients, should bring and use their own devices, and not be limited to the use of pre-configured and unfamiliar devices. The BYOD concept has been successfully implemented various educational and industrial context. BYOD is less frequent in e-Health, but as highlighted in the study by Brooks (2014), BYOD could be a valuable complement to traditional healthcare and rehabilitation.

5   Conclusion

The study has established some important requirements for further testing on a planned group of patients. Firstly, the general requirements for overall technology-enhanced stroke rehabilitation are investigated and then specific requirements for three established categories, cognitive, motoric and speech rehabilitation after stroke are explored.

Technology-enhanced systems seem to have various benefits that can support independent living and increase the quality of life of a stroke survivor. However, a user-centered approach is essential to design these TES where user-friendliness and usefulness plays an important role in the success of TES. Stroke patients often suffer from different kind/degree of mental and physical disabilities such as memory loss and visual deficiency, therefore, TES should be adopted according to the patient's current medical condition. Patients' close relatives and friends can also play a vital role in the success of TES, therefore, they should also be involved in the technology-enhanced rehabilitation process. The study findings contributed significantly in the Mid Sweden region since the population is scattered in the whole region and TES can provide batter and equal treatment possibilities in the remote areas of the region.

6   Future Research

The identified need for taylormade rehabilitation software requires further studies. An interesting idea would be to design, develop and evaluate a software prototype based on the requirements that have been gathered in this study. The prototype design should also be revised and updated according to the results of a continuous user test starting very early in the process.

References

Ahmad, A., Mozelius, P., Ahlin, K.: Testbed requirements for technology enhanced stroke rehabilitation to support independent living. In: ICT4AWE 2019-5th International Conference on Information and Communication Technologies for Ageing Well and e-Health, Heraklion, Greece, pp. 174–182 INSTICC Press, 2–4 May 2019

Alankus, G., Lazar, A., May, M., Kelleher, C.: Towards customizable games for stroke rehabilitation. In: Proceedings of the SIGCHI Conference on Human Factors in Computing Systems, pp. 2113–2122. ACM (2010)

Almborg, A.H., Ulander, K., Thulin, A., Berg, S.: Discharge planning of stroke patients: the relatives' perceptions of participation. J. Clin. Nurs. **18**(6), pp. 857–865 (2009)

Arntzen, C., Hamran, T.: Stroke survivors' and relatives' negotiation of relational and activity changes: a qualitative study. Scand. J. Occup. Therapy **23**(1), 39–49 (2016)

Bengtsson, M.: How to plan and perform a qualitative study using content analysis. NursingPlus Open **2**, 8–14 (2016)

Boian, R., et al.: Virtual reality-based post-stroke hand rehabilitation. Stud. Health Technol. Inform. 64–70 (2002)

Brady, M.C., Kelly, H., Godwin, J., Enderby, P., Campbell, P.: Speech and language therapy for aphasia following stroke. Cochrane Database Syst. Rev. 6, 323-351 (2016). Art. No.: CD000425. https://doi.org/10.1002/14651858.cd000425.pub4

Brooks, A.L.: Disruptive innovation in healthcare and rehabilitation. In: Brooks, A., Brahnam, S., Jain, L. (eds.) Technologies of Inclusive Well-Being, vol. 536. Springer, Heidelberg (2014). https://doi.org/10.1007/978-3-642-45432-5_16

Burke, J.W., McNeill, M.D.J., Charles, D.K., Morrow, P.J., Crosbie, J.H., McDonough, S.M.: Optimising engagement for stroke rehabilitation using serious games. Vis. Comput. **25**(12), 1085 (2009)

Choi, Y.H., Ku, J., Lim, H., Kim, Y.H., Paik, N.J.: Mobile game-based virtual reality rehabilitation program for upper limb dysfunction after ischemic stroke. Restorative Neurol. Neurosci. **34**(3), 455–463 (2016)

Cogollor, J.M., et al.: Evolution of cognitive rehabilitation after stroke from traditional techniques to smart and personalized home-based information and communication technology systems: literature review. JMIR Rehabil. Assist. Technol. **5**(1), e4 (2018)

Dabbs, A.D.V., et al.: User-centered design and interactive health technologies for patients. Comput. Inform. Nurs.: CIN **27**(3), 175 (2009)

Dahlbom, B., Mathiassen, L.: A Scandinavian view on ACM's code of ethics (2017). https://doi.org/10.1145/181900.181902

Dimaguila, G.L., Gray, K., Merolli, M.: Person-generated health data in simulated rehabilitation using Kinect for stroke: literature review. JMIR Rehabil. Assist. Technol. **5**(1), e11 (2018)

Elo, S., Kyngäs, H.: The qualitative content analysis process. J. Adv. Nurs. **62**, 107–115 (2008)

Erlingsson, C., Brysiewicz, P.: A hands-on guide to doing content analysis. Afr. J. Emerg. Med. **7**, 93-99 (2017)

Gamito, P., et al.: Cognitive training on stroke patients via virtual reality-based serious games. Disability Rehabil. **39**(4), 385–388 (2017)

Gerstenecker, A., Lazar, R.M.: Language recovery following stroke. Clin. Neuropsychol. 1-20 (2019)

Glasgow, R.E.: eHealth evaluation and dissemination research. Am. J. Prevent. Med. **32**(5), S119–S126 (2007)

Gwozdz, W., Sousa-Poza, A.: Ageing, health and life satisfaction of the oldest old: an analysis for Germany. Soc. Indic. Res. **97**(3), 397–417 (2010)

Helgesson, G.: Forskningsetik (Andra upplagan). Studentlitteratur, Lund (2015). Hong, T.: Discourses on honour-related violence in finnish policy documents. NORA-Nordic J. Feminist Gend. Res. **22**(4), 314–329 (2014)

Heruti, R.J., et al.: Rehabilitation outcome of elderly patients after a first stroke: effect of cognitive status at admission on the functional outcome. Arch. Phys. Med. Rehabil. **83**(6), 742–749 (2002)

Hevner, A.R., March, S.T., Park, J., Ram, S.: Design science in information systems research. MIS Q. **28**(1), 75–105 (2004)

Hilari, K., Wiggins, R., Roy, P., Byng, S., Smith, S.: Predictors of health-related quality of life (HRQL) in people with chronic aphasia. Aphasiology **17**(4), pp. 365–381 (2003)

Johannesson, P., Perjons, E.: An Introduction to Design Science. Springer, Heidelberg (2014). https://doi.org/10.1007/978-3-319-10632-8

Johansson, M.B., Carlsson, M., Sonnander, K.: Communication difficulties and the use of communication strategies: from the perspective of individuals with aphasia. Int. J. Lang. Commun. Disorders **47**(2), 144–155 (2012)

Jokinen, H., et al.: Post-stroke cognitive impairment is common even after successful clinical recovery. Eur. J. Neurol. **22**(9), 1288–1294 (2015)

Juul, J.: A Casual Revolution: Reinventing Video Games and Their Players. MIT Press, Cambridge (2010)

Kesav, P., Vrinda, S., Sukumaran, S., Sarma, P., Sylaja, P.: Effectiveness of speech language therapy either alone or with add-on computer-based language therapy software (Malayalam version) for early post stroke aphasia: a feasibility study'. J. Neurol. Sci. **380**, 137–141 (2017)

Kvale, S., Brinkmann, S.: Den kvalitativa forskningsintervjun. Studentlitteratur, Lund (2014)

Langhorne, P., Coupar, F., Pollock, A.: Motor recovery after stroke: a systematic review. Lancet Neurol. **8**(8), 741–754 (2009)

Langhorne, P., Bernhardt, J., Kwakkel, G.: Stroke rehabilitation. Lancet **377**(9778), 1693–1702 (2011)

Lomer, M., McLellan, D.L.: Informing hospital patients and their relatives about stroke. Clin. Rehabil. **1**(1), 33–37 (1987)

Mallet, K., et al.: RecoverNow: a patient perspective on the delivery of mobile tablet-based stroke rehabilitation in the acute care setting. Int. J. Stroke **14**(2), 174–179 (2019)

Neuhauser, L., Kreps, G.L., Morrison, K., Athanasoulis, M., Kirienko, N., Van Brunt, D.: Using design science and artificial intelligence to improve health communication: ChronologyMD case example. Patient Educ. Counseling **92**(2), 211–217 (2013)

Nicolau, H., Guerreiro, T., Pereira, R., Gonçalves, D., Jorge, J.: Computer-assisted rehabilitation: towards effective evaluation. Int. J. Cogn. Performance Support **1**(1), 11–26 (2013)

Orihuela-Espina, F., et al.: Robot training for hand motor recovery in subacute stroke patients: a randomized controlled trial. J. Hand Therapy **29**(1), 51–57 (2016)

Pastorino, M., et al.: Preliminary evaluation of a personal healthcare system prototype for cognitive eRehabilitation in a living assistance domain. Sensors **14**(6), 10213–10233 (2014)

Pagliari, C.: Design and evaluation in eHealth: challenges and implications for an interdisciplinary field. J. Med. Internet Res. **9**(2), e15 (2007)

Palmcrantz, S., et al.: An interactive distance solution for stroke rehabilitation in the home setting–a feasibility study. Inform. Health Soc. Care **42**(3), 303-320 (2017)

Parker, J., Mawson, S.: Providing sources of self-efficacy through technology enhanced post-stroke rehabilitation in the home. In: AAATE Conference, pp. 401-408 (2017)

Peek, S.T., et al.: Older adults' reasons for using technology while aging in place. Gerontology **62**(2), 226–237 (2016)

Peel, N., Bartlett, H., McClure, R.: Healthy ageing: how is it defined and measured? Australas. J. Ageing **23**(3), 115–119 (2004)

Peffers, K., Tuunanen, T., Rothenberger, M.A., Chatterjee, S.: A design science research methodology for information systems research. J. Manag. Inf. Syst. **24**(3), 45–77 (2007)

Pollock, A., et al.: Physical rehabilitation approaches for the recovery of function and mobility following stroke. Cochrane Database Syst. Rev. (4) (2014)

Ross, K., Wertz, R.: Quality of life with and without aphasia. Aphasiology 17(4), 355–364 (2003)

Rybarczyk, Y., Fonseca, J.: Tangible interface for a rehabilitation of comprehension in aphasic patients (2011)

Rybarczyk, Y., Fonseca, J., Martins, R.: Lisling 3D: a serious game for the treatment of Portuguese aphasic patients. In: Proceedings of 12th Conference of the Association for the Advancement of Assistive Technology in Europe (2013)

Simic, T., Leonard, C., Laird, L., Cupit, J., Höbler, F., Rochon, E.: A usability study of internet-based therapy for naming deficits in aphasia. Am. J. Speech Lang. Pathol. 25(4), 642–653 (2016)

Skidmore, E.R., et al.: Cognitive and affective predictors of rehabilitation participation after stroke. Arch. Phys. Med. Rehabil. 91(2), 203–207 (2010)

Stinear, C.M., Byblow, W.D.: Predicting and accelerating motor recovery after stroke. Curr. Opin. Neurol. 27(6), 624–630 (2014)

Tousignant, M., et al.: Satisfaction with in-home speech telerehabilitation in post-stroke aphasia: an exploratory analysis. J. Int. Soc. Telemed. eHealth 6, e11 (11–18) (2018)

Veerbeek, J.M., et al.: What is the evidence for physical therapy poststroke? A systematic review and meta-analysis. PloS One 9(2), e87987 (2014)

Vourvopoulos, A., Faria, A.L., Cameirao, M.S., i Badia, S.B.: RehabNet: a distributed architecture for motor and cognitive neuro-rehabilitation. In: 2013 IEEE 15th International Conference on e-Health Networking, Applications and Services, pp. 454-459. IEEE (2013)

Wade, E., Winstein, C.J.: Virtual reality and robotics for stroke rehabilitation: where do we go from here? Topics Stroke Rehabil. 18(6), 685–700 (2011)

Wieringa, R.J.: Design Science Methodology for Information Systems and Software Engineering. Springer, Heidelberg (2014). https://doi.org/10.1007/978-3-662-43839-8

Øra, H.P., Kirmess, M., Brady, M.C., Winsnes, I.E., Hansen, S.M., Becker, F.: Telerehabilitation for aphasia protocol of a pragmatic, exploratory, pilot randomized controlled trial. Trials 19(1), 208 (2018)

Zhang, H., Shen, Z., Lin, J., Chen, Y., Miao, Y.: Familiarity design in exercise games for elderly. Int. J. Inf. Technol. 22, 1–19 (2016)

Evaluating iTV Companion Application with Seniors

Telmo Silva[1,2(✉)] and Martinho Mota[1,2]

[1] Digimedia, Department of Communication and Arts, University of Aveiro, Aveiro, Portugal
{tsilva,m.vaz.mota}@ua.pt
[2] Campus Universitário de Santiago, 3810-193 Aveiro, Portugal

Abstract. Technological advances are contributing to higher levels of quality of life in developed countries, as new solutions emerge at an increasing speed, quantity, and quality to answer the population's lifestyle needs and desires. Seniors nowadays constitute a significant portion of the world population and thus, concerns in answer to their needs are becoming more common from the governments and enterprises' side taking technological resources into account. In this context, this paper presents the results of testing a second-screen mobile application designed for senior users. The work presented in this paper was carried out under the +TV4E project, which aims to promote the info-inclusion of Portuguese senior population by sending them information about public and social services. The mobile application described here is part of the project and is a second-screen approach of the already existing iTV application that delivers informative videos to seniors. The mobile app also allows users to access their videos but in a more flexible way. The development process was composed of four major phases: i) prototype development; ii) tests with a small set of seniors; iii) prototype enhancement; iv) Tests in a real context of use.

Keywords: Seniors · iTV · Mobile applications · Companion applications · Second-screen applications · Usability · User experience

1 Introduction

Population aging is an inevitable natural occurrence that has led to a significant inversion of the aging pyramid in the developed societies in the last decades. Nearly every country is facing an increased longevity of adults, which in turn reflect in an increase of older people, both in the number and proportions [1]. This phenomenon became one of the greatest challenges for modern civilization and is affecting all sectors of society, namely labor and financial markets, goods and services, such as housing, transportation and social protection [2]. Forecasts indicate that a rapid increase in the number of people aged 60 or over in the medium-term will occur in the near future. Between 2015 and 2030 it is estimated that the total population aged 60 years and over will increase from 901 million to 1.4 billion, reaching nearly 2.1 billion in 2050 [2]. This increase in life expectancy can be considered as a great achievement for developed societies, however, it raises various challenges and concerns to citizens, governments, and communities.

M. Ziefle and L. A. Maciaszek (Eds.): ICT4AWE 2019, CCIS 1219, pp. 160–179, 2020.
https://doi.org/10.1007/978-3-030-52677-1_9

Changes in public health policies, retirement and pension policies, social security and education, are some of the consequences of demographic aging [3, 4]. Although aging is characterized by several physical, psychological and social changes which can result in various problems, being old does not necessarily have to be synonymous of illness, disability, dependency, isolation, or loneliness. Living longer can become distressing and problematic for both the individuals themselves and for those around them when proper conditions for being independent, active, and healthy are not available. It is important to develop policies and strategies that allow older people to maintain or improve their quality of life so that aging start being seen from the perspective of "add life to years" instead of "add years to life". Considering the aging process, the concept of "quality of life" is highly determined by the individual's ability to maintain their autonomy and independence [5].

Particularly in Portugal, 2,032,606 citizens were 65 years or over in 2012. Considering optimistic projections and the current trends of fertility, mortality and migration, in 2060 this number will increase to 3,343,987 [6]. Information is vital for everyone, especially the senior population, which needs to stay well informed so that they can adapt their lifestyle within social and governmental norms, maintaining their autonomy and independence. Access to information is one of the areas which influence seniors' quality of life the most. It allows people to be more knowledgeable about their environments and thus allow them to make decisions in a more supported manner [7]. In Portugal, despite the existence of plenty of information regarding social and public services, which is made available in several service outlets as well as online platforms, often seniors cannot easily access it because it requires a certain degree of proficiency in technical terms which can be hard to understand by most of the citizens. To further aggravate this situation for the senior population, accessing this information involves a pro-active behavior by the user, often not seen in seniors [8].

In this context, the +TV4E platform's goal is to bring information regarding social and public services to seniors, allowing them to easily gain access to services without the need to search for them. The core of this platform consists in notifying users of informative content about social or public services while they watch TV. Not to lose any television content, the platforms allows the seniors to automatically pause the TV broadcast to watch an informative video and then continue watching the linear broadcast. These informative videos are divided into seven areas of general interest named ASGIE [9], which include Healthcare and Welfare services, Social services, Financial services, Culture services, Security services, Transport services and Local authority services. In addition, the +TV4E platform features a video library which aggregates every informative video sent to the user and a video recommendation algorithm, used to determine which videos should be sent to each user. The project intends to offer seniors an easier way to access information about public and social services, contributing to a more independent way of living. This project was developed in collaboration with several groups of seniors who took part in iterative design sessions and usability tests, to evaluate a high-fidelity prototype of the product.

2 Aging and Mobile Interfaces

It is important for seniors to be included in a society that is constantly evolving considering the challenges related to the aging process and the characteristics of older people themselves. Considering this need, the term active aging emerged and was adopted in 2002 by the World Health Organization. The organization advocated that in order for older people to maintain a good quality of life, a lengthier lifespan must be accompanied by continuous opportunities in health, security, and participation. These three concepts are defined as the pillars of what constitutes active aging and encourages individuals, throughout their life course, to realize their potential for physical, social, and mental wellbeing and to participate in society, while providing them the adequate protection, security, and care, when needed [5, 10]. During the aging process, the quality of life depends on the risks and opportunities experienced over life course. As far as the persons get old, the support provided by other generations is from capital importance. [5]. An active aging process allows people to keep their sense of purpose and belonging after they become retired, disabled or incapacitated, encouraging them to play an active role in their respective families, communities, and social groups. This approach followed by the World Health Organization has based the recognition of senior's human rights and the principles of independence, participation, dignity, care, and self-realization defined by the United Nations [11]. This concept allows the recognition of aging as a global phenomenon, encouraging people to work for longer and to retire later or to engage in volunteer work after retirement, thus maintaining healthy and independent lives [10]. But this recognition will also create new challenges to public health systems to ensure that seniors continue to have access to means that allow them to age in a healthy and autonomous way [1]. In this context, technologies play an important role providing senior population with several benefits, helping them to maintain a higher quality of life for longer. Nowadays, we are constantly facing the appearance of innovative technologies in a widespread of fields such as medicine, robotics, assisted living mediated by sensors [1]. However, developing technologies for seniors can become a tricky process because, ultimately, their adoption relies on the senior's capacity to understand and adapt to them [10]. It is important to never forget that this audience may have low levels of digital literacy and therefore can be less prepared to handle complex digital tasks, so these technologies need to be adapted to seniors instead of forcing seniors to adapt to them.

When developing solutions for seniors designers should be aware that they need to accommodate all the physiological changes that occur with aging, which cause the need for a higher degree of support in executing tasks and activities [12]. Neglecting seniors' accessibility issues on the application's design process alongside the fact is often hard for them to get used to new technologies are the main causes for the low levels of technology acceptance [13]. In 2006, Hawthorn highlights in his investigation "Designing Effective Interfaces for Older Users" [14], that despite his users having ages between 65 and 85 years old, their numeric age was somewhat insignificant [10]. The key factors influencing interface design are related to the aging process itself thus influencing the as loss of vision and memory, as well as the decrease in learning speed. Pereira in [15] states that most of digital interfaces are not designed considering the sensory, physical and cognitive constraints of seniors. Loss of hearing and visual acuity, for example, are factors that need to be considered when developing software for seniors. Reis and colleges [16] provide a set of guidelines to ensure technology' acceptance by senior users. The visual acuity problems commonly associated with seniors' causes them to have difficulty in focusing at short distances, distinguishing small details, discriminating chromatic differences and reading moving text. Additionally, it lowers their adaptability to lighting making them more susceptible to brightness variations and thus requiring, for example a in a more luminous space for reading. To overcome these visual limitation there are various guidelines that should be considered to ensure that the software is designed appropriately. Guidelines suggest that the onscreen text should be at least 40pts, the fonts should not have serifs, italic or other decorative elements, the text should be aligned to the left, the spacing between lines needs to guarantee fluidity and readability and there should be high contrast between the background and the text [16]. Titles and labels should be large and easy to read. Regarding iconography, icons should be easily distinguishable, the use of abstract concepts or any current graphical conventions associated with the ICT should be avoided and most importantly, as a failsafe, be composed of a combination of text plus an image, where the text helps reinforce the meaning of the icon [10, 16]. The colors are also another important aspect to consider and should be chosen carefully to account for the limited colors spectrum seniors perceive and the fact that colors never look alike in different screens. Physical challenges of using technology, skeptical attitudes regarding the benefits of technology, complex security settings and even the complexity of basic online services related with social security, finances, or health services emerge as potentially dissuasion factors for the use of ICT by seniors. To some extent, this situation may contribute to the seniors' info exclusion [17].

When working on strategies designed to promote the access of information by seniors, it is important to understand them and be aware of their information consumption habits. With these concepts in mind, the project +TV4E provides users of the platform with an alternative way of consuming information with the addition of a mobile application. The platform was initially designed for the TV as a medium of delivering informative content regarding social and public services to seniors. In this paper the inclusion of a mobile application in the +TV4E ecosystem is described. This mobile application aims to further expand the effectiveness of the +TV4E platform in delivering information using a mobile companion application and thus better serve the needs of seniors.

3   Design and Development of the Mobile Companion Application

The design and development of the mobile application was divided into three phases: i) the definition of the functional and technical requirements, ii) the design of the interface and iii) the implementation. Defining the functional requirements, was arguably the most important step in this process, since, it was necessary to find a balance between the iTV and the mobile application to serve as a complement and not a replacement to the +TV4E iTV solution. The mobile application was planned to take advantage of the functionalities available on smartphones (having a keyboard, which allows for easier typing, touch controls, a microphone, a camera and most importantly being portable) to enhance the potential of the iTV +TV4E solution. The following set of functional requirements was defined [10]:

a) Scan QR codes for a simplified user login
b) Allow the user to access his/her video library
c) Enable the user to watch informative videos on the smartphone
d) Allow the user to select a video and watch it on the TV
e) Allow the user to search videos on his/her video library
f) Provide the user with recommended videos for his profile
g) Allow the user to use voice commands to interact with the TV
h) Include a tutorial to help the users

The +TV4E mobile application was designed to work both: i) as a second-screen application, for when the user is watching TV at home and ii) as a standalone application to watch informative videos outside. So the application would allow the user to browse his personal video library anywhere, thus being fully a functional way to watch informative videos when he's away from the TV, but also allow the user to interact with the TV by using the application to search for and push videos to the TV [10]. Alongside with the functional requirements it were defined the technical requirements of the +TV4E mobile application that are listed below [10]:

a) Run on Android smartphones
b) Be able to communicate with the set-top box
c) Be able to access the internet
d) Be able to access the smartphone's camera and microphone
e) Feature touch controls

In the time frame of this work, it was impossible to develop for both Android and iOS. In this context, it was decided to develop to the Android platform taking advantage from iOS either the application needs to be published in the app store or the device needs to be configured to allow the installation of unverified applications. Furthermore, Android devices are vastly more common thus facilitating the gathering of participants to test the application.

The development of the application considered also that the mobile application should be able to directly communicate with the set-top box in order to function as a companion application for when the user is watching TV, as well as connect to the internet in order to stream the informative videos, access the smartphone's microphone to record the user's voice during voice commands and the smartphone's camera to scan the QR codes that identify uniquely the user' set-top box.

After establishing the requirements the design process of the interface began keeping in mind that the layout should be as simple as possible while accommodating all the features in a clear and visible way. Simplicity was the focus since familiarity with technology usually decreases with age and seniors tend to avoid technology when the product is too complicated for them. Individual abilities decline with old age, especially vision, since the eyes lose its ability to focus quickly or to react to rapidly-changing brightness it is important to accommodate these limitations in the design. Seniors often also cannot see thin lines or other fine details in interfaces and have difficulty distinguishing between similar icons, therefore, the interface was kept as clean and simple as possible consisting only of two main screens ("Library" and "Recommendations") the login screen, a menu, a tutorial and a total of only three icons. The "Library" screen aggregates all the videos sent to the user in the last 15 days in a vertical list ordered by the most recent, each video is presented as a card, similarly to the Youtube™ mobile application, containing the title, the duration, the date it was sent and a thumbnail representing the area of interest of the video. By clicking on the card, the user is shown an on-screen prompt which asks him if he wants to watch the video on the smartphone or the TV. Additionally, this screen contains a search bar which allows the user to find videos by their title which is represented by a magnifying glass icon. The "Recommendations" screen follows the same layout of the previous screen, however, it displays a maximum of six videos suggested by the + TV4E recommendation system and it does not feature a search bar since the video list is much smaller. To implement the login in a simplified manner a QR code was added to the set-top boxes which contained the serial number of the box, this way if a user needed to login in the mobile application he would only have to scan the QR code located on top of the box, thus removing the need to remember a username and password combination. The menu was positioned at the top of the screen, to avoid having the user accidentally clicking on it while scrolling, and featured two buttons which served both as shortcuts to navigate between the two main screens and to let the user know which screen he was navigating since the selected screen was highlighted. Finally, on the bottom right of the screen, two buttons were positioned, the "Help" button was represented by a question mark icon and opened the tutorial and the "Voice" button allowed the user to issue a voice commands to the ITV application. Figure 1 depicts the basic navigation flow.

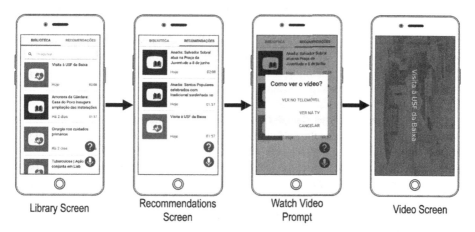

| Library Screen | Recommendations Screen | Watch Video Prompt | Video Screen |

Fig. 1. Prototype screens [10].

In order to optimize the skills of developers (they were used to developing Javascript web applications) it was chosen Ionic framework Ionic to develop the mobile application, an open-source software development kit built on AngularJS, allowing the development of hybrid mobile applications using web technologies such as HTLM5 and CSS. The development followed the specifications stated previously, with the two main screens and a tutorial area, the voice commands were implemented using Google's Speech to Text service and the interaction with the set-top box was done by sending HTTP requests to the +TV4E web API which then communicated with the box via a socket connection [10, 18].

In the next section, the methodology used to evaluate the mobile application is described in detail, going over the objectives of the study, the sample, and the testing process.

4 Testing Methodology

This paper depicts the inclusion of a mobile companion application and assess its added value in the already existing +TV4E platform. To accomplish this objective, firstly it is necessary to evaluate the Usability and User experience of the developed application. To evaluate these aspects, it is necessary to decide a set of scales that can provide accurate results in assessing the usability and the user-experience, as well as being appropriate to be applied with the target demographic. The present section describes this process, going over the objective, the sample and detailing the entire process.

4.1 Goals

The main goal of this testing procedure was to evaluate the usability and user-experience of the +TV4E mobile application, which would serve as a companion of the iTV application developed under the +TV4E project. The idea of the application was from the research team, rather than being an idea proposed by seniors during the participatory design sessions of the +TV4E project. Despite and considering the literature (that strongly suggests that the best way to develop software solutions for the senior population is to work closely with them) seniors' opinion was considered along with all the development process. By engaging with seniors in key development steps it is easier to create a solution that better suits the needs of this population, which often has difficulties handling newer technologies.

In terms of functionalities, The +TV4E mobile application serves a similar purpose to the video library present in the iTV application, which allows users to watch videos on-demand, thus giving some control over which content the users want to see, as opposed to the way videos are automatically sent to users while watching the regular television broadcast in the ITV Application [18]. In both the library and the mobile application, the users can re-watch videos they already saw or catch up on videos they missed or ignored while watching TV, however in the latter the users are given a higher degree of control since they can also watch suggested videos based on their usage of the platform. These suggested videos are provided by the recommendation system, which is also used when choosing which video should be sent to each user [19]. Additionally, the mobile application provides the users with a search feature, allowing them to watch videos either on their smartphones or in the TV and also to interact with the iTV application via voice commands. These commands allow the user to perform a very limited amount of actions, namely selecting the next higher or lower channel, changing to a specific TV channel given its name or number, and accessing the video library. This feature was implemented due to the rising popularity of voice assistants in the market, such as Siri, Alexa and Google Assistant, which made the research team consider including them in the mobile application in order to assess how the senior population would react to them in a TV ecosystem.

However similar in terms of functionality, the mobile application greatly differs from the video library when it comes to its interface and user experience especially since it is developed on for a different platform with a significantly different interaction paradigm, therefore the need to perform new tests to validate it with seniors. The key elements in need of validation were the navigation, the interface, the voice commands and the general receptiveness for this technology to be integrated into the +TV4E platform [10].

4.2 Participants

The sample for this study was divided into two groups, a first group to perform a preliminary usability analysis, which aimed at finding key usability issues in the application [20], and a second group to test the application in a real home environment with the full +TV4E platform.

The first sample group was composed of five individuals of the Senior University of Curia, four females (80%) and one male (20%), with an average age of 71.4 years, four of these individuals completed a higher education degree while the fifth only completed middle school. The only requirements to participate in this sample were being at least 60 years old, having a basic knowledge on how to use a smartphone since the application was being designed for users who already use a smartphone on a daily basis, and being familiar with the +TV4E project. This sample was inquired regarding their smartphone usage, none of them required help while using their smartphones, four users (80%) used an Android device while one (20%) used an iOS device and the average time spent user their phone per day was 1.1 h. Lastly, the participants were asked about which actions they perform using their smartphones, the results are depicted in the following table (Table 1):

Table 1. Smartphone usage for the first sample group [10].

Smartphone usage	n	%
(1) Making phone calls	5	100
(2) Sending text messages	5	100
(3) Reading news	3	60
(4) Using social networks	2	40
(5) Play games	1	20

As expected all users use their smartphones to make phones calls and send text messages, however the more advanced features, which require a higher level of proficiency, were less prevalent in this sample.

The second sample group included four senior participants, three females (60%) and two males (40%), with an average age of 67.2 years, the average education level of this sample was lower with three (60%) of these individuals completed primary and two (40%) of them completed middle school. The requirements for this sample were the same as the previous group, being over 60 years old and knowing how to use a smartphone, except that it was not required for them to already be familiar with the + TV4E project since this group was going to test the entire platform. The participants of this sample reported that they used their smartphones for an average of 2.8 hours per day, 80% of them were Android users while only 20% were iOS users and actions they reported to perform on their smartphones are shown in the following table (Table 2):

Table 2. Smartphone usage for the second sample group.

Smartphone usage	n	%
(1) Making phone calls	5	100
(2) Sending text messages	5	100
(3) Reading news	4	80
(4) Using social networks	4	80
(5) Play games	0	0

Similarly, to the previous sample group, every participant stated that they use their smartphones to make phone calls and send text messages, however, this group displayed higher usage of the more advanced features, specifically browsing news and using social network applications.

4.3 Tests with Users

After the design and development process was concluded, the next step was the evaluation of the mobile application's first prototype in a controlled environment with a small sample of five users to find the major flaws in its design. To accomplish this, the application was presented to the first sample group composed of students of the Senior University of Curia. The first testing phase was divided into two parts, initially, the application was presented to each participant which then tested it individually during a cognitive walkthrough and then all the participants were gathered to discuss their experiences in a focus group. After this phase, various improvements were made in the mobile application considering the data gathered with the first sample group. Finally, the second phase was conducted in the homes of the second sample group and consisted of user tests in a real context of use using the entire +TV4E platform, being followed by interviews and a focus group in the end. The entire process is depicted in Fig. 2 and each of these steps will be described in greater detail in the following sections.

Controlled Environment Tests. The first phase of tests began by contextualizing the participants regarding the test they were about to take part in, reminding them about the +TV4E project (explaning the core idea and remembering the main funcionalities),

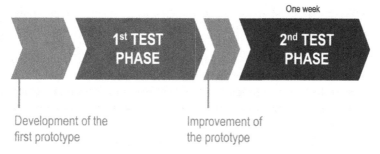

Fig. 2. Mobile application test phases [10].

since all of them took part in previous data gatherings, explaining that their participation was voluntary and that the data collected would remain anonymous and would not be disclosed. Afterward, the participants signed the informed consent to take part in the study and their demographic data was collected, the participants were asked their age, gender and level of education, followed by a survey regarding their smartphone usage habits, on which they were asked what device they use, their daily average use and which tasks they perform regularly with the smartphone (the results of this survey were already presented in a previous section).

Next, each participant was given a brief explanation of the mobile application's features, emphasizing the fact that it mostly consisted of a complement to the iTV application they tested previously. Then they took part in a cognitive walkthrough composed of 14 tasks which aimed at evaluating key aspects of the interface and layout of the application. The tasks were the following:

1. Open the +TV4E mobile application
2. Read the application's user guide
3. Login to the application using the provided QR code
4. Access the help menu and review the application's user guide
5. Count the number of videos in the list "My Videos"
6. Point out when the 3rd video of the list was added
7. Use the search function to search for the video "USF Almada"
8. Watch on the smartphone the video you searched
9. Close the video you are watching
10. Switch to the list "Recommended Videos"
11. Point out the duration of the 2nd video in the list
12. Chose a video from the list and watch it on the television
13. Click on the microphone button and use a voice command to change the TV channel
14. Use a voice command to access the video library

During the execution of these tasks, a performance evaluation chart was filled out registering whether the task was successfully completed, the number of mistakes, the execution time and other usage details. The participants were encouraged to perform the tasks independently, thus the researcher gave as little instructions as possible and instead just motivated them to keep trying. However, if the participant decided to give up it the solution would be explained to him while he explained why he could not finish the task since some tasks required the completion of previous ones. After concluding the tasks, the participants were asked to fill out a Self-Assessment Manikin test.

The test process allowed each participant to test the application individually. Then all participants participated in a focus group where they were encouraged to discuss which aspects of the mobile application they considered to need improvements, which features should be included to this initial prototype and if they found the application useful or not. The focus group was structured to center the discussion around these three aspects and included a set of open-ended questions [10]. All the participants were given an opportunity to express their opinions as well as discuss among themselves their user experience, this step was considered crucial for this early testing since it provided a very direct feedback of the main problems found in the application at the moment.

Before the second test phase, all the data gathered was compiled and used to identify the most recurring problems in the application. Using this results the layout was improved in order to better suit the target audience needs.

The majority of these issues were obtained through direct user feedback while some of them were inferred by the research team, they were divided into three categories: i) issues reported directly by the users, ii) issues identified by the researcher during the user testing and iii) software issues. Among the user reported problems, the most frequent issue, which occurred in all user tests, was the fact the users were assuming that the duration of the video was instead the time at which it was added. The majority of users complained also that it was difficult for them to exit a video they were watching, so a button was added to the top right corner of the screen with the label "exit" which would only appear while a video was being played. Also, regarding the video player, it was decided to remove the player controls and only keep the play/pause function by tapping the screen since the users frequently clicked on the timeline by accident. The contrast of the colors was slightly altered to allow for better legibility since some users complained it was too bright to read. Regarding the buttons, since most users found it difficult to understand the chosen iconography for the "Help" and "Microphone" buttons, labels were added to them to avoid confusion. Additionally, the overall size of all buttons was increased since most users expressed difficulty in pressing them.

By observation of the tests it was made clear that a search bar should also be present in the "Recommended Videos" list both for consistency and for times when there are several recommended videos. As far as the tutorial was considered not to be very useful since it lacked clear instructions on how to use the application's features, the team updated it to include close-ups of each function and text clearly explaining each one [10]. Regarding technical problems, the development team identified some: i) the search bar did not update when the user pressed the backspace and ii) the "Microphone" button was not properly requesting permission to access the smartphone's microphone, needed for the voice commands.

All the identified issues during this test phase were fixed leading to the second prototype of the +TV4E mobile application. This allowed the research team to make a second phase to the mobile application.

Field Trial. The second and final phase of testing lasted for 8 days, during which the second sample group took part in a field test in their own homes using the entire +TV4E platform. Similarly to the previous phase, the objectives of the test were explained to the participants, they were asked to sign off an informed consent and provided the same demographic data collected from the previous sample group. Afterward, the research team installed the necessary equipment for testing the platform, which involved hooking up the set-top box to a TV, installing a 4G router to guarantee a stable internet connection and finally installing the mobile application in the participant's smartphone.

After explaining how the platform worked, especially how the mobile application worked in tandem with the ITV application, the users were left to test it for a total of eight days, during this period the research team kept regular contact with the participants to ensure the system was working properly and provide support if necessary. During this time the system was keeping records of the videos each user watched, it registered when the video was seen, which method was used for watching the video, either via notification, library or the mobile application and the rating given at the end of the video.

On the last day of testing, before removing the equipment from the user's homes, each user was interviewed regarding their experience using the +TV4E platform. These were semi-structured interviews where the participant was encouraged to share any aspects they either liked or disliked regarding the mobile application and afterward they were asked the same set questions used in the previous focus group for the sake of having some consistency in the results.

The final step was conducting a focus group in a similar fashion to the previous phase, where all the participants who just tested the platform were gathered and asked to discuss their experiences during the past eight days. This was a structured focus group and included the following open-ended questions:

1. How did you feel while testing the +TV4E platform?
2. What made watch a notified video or searching for a video on the mobile application
3. During the interviews I understood that you rather use the platform on the television, why is that?
4. In your opinion which device is easier to use, the ITV or the mobile application?
5. In your opinion what are the main positive and negative aspects of ITV application? And of the mobile application?
6. Do you have suggestions to improve the ITV or the mobile applications in order to make it more accessible to seniors?

This focus group was aimed at comparing the ITV application with the mobile application, which was something being studied in parallel with the interface and user-experience evaluation of the mobile application, therefore only the answers to the last two questions were relevant for this study and are going to be later considered in the final results.

5   Results Analysis

A total of 10 individuals took part in this study which spawned across two testing phases, during which two versions of the mobile application were tested. The results of these tests are divided into each of the phases and further by each testing method applied.

5.1   Controlled Environment

The first phase, composed by a cognitive walkthrough, a user experience questioner (SAM) and a focus group, allowed to evaluate the first prototype of the mobile application.

During the tests in the controlled environment it was performed a cognitive walkthrough test allowing verify the main issues concerning the mobile application interface design [10].

Looking at the results of the cognitive walkthrough, out of the 14 tasks only 5 were not successfully completed by all the users. Task 1 (Open the +TV4E mobile application) proved to be problematic mainly due to two reasons: two users complained the icon was not easy to identify while a third had problems since she was an iOS user and therefore was not used to Android smartphones. The task "Read the application's user guide" had a high rate of success, but four users had some trouble understanding they needed to swipe right to advance the tutorial. All users completed the task "Login to the application using the provided QR code" contrary to the expectations. Since the process was compared to taking a photo with the smartphone, the users easily carried out the task. Task 4 (Access the help menu and review the application's user guide) displayed the lowest success rate since three of the five users could not identify the question mark icon as being the help button. Task 7 (Use the search function to search for the video "USF Almada") was hard to complete by three users because they had difficulty typing the title of the requested video, this can be due to the smartphone used for testing being different to the devices the users are used to type with. The users had no difficulty in closing the video they are watching, however, the average execution time was higher than expected since exiting the video should be a simple task, users reported that using the smartphone's back button was not an intuitive way to exit the video since not all smartphones have a back button and sometimes the button is swapped with the overview button. Finally, concerning the tasks related with voice commands ("Click on the microphone button and use a voice command to change the TV channel" and "Use a voice command to access the video library") all the users completed them without any issues and with the lowest execution time .

Finished the cognitive walkthrough a SAM questionnaire was applied. This evaluation tool focuses on three items, namely pleasure, arousal, and dominance.

Analyzing the results, it is clear that, the users rated the application highly on all three items, arousal and pleasure were especially high, which can be attributed to the fact that the users where testing technologies that are still relatively new to them, especially the voice commands, which all five users later reported to find very interesting. However, the lowest score in dominance was the main take away from this SAM, which cannot be dismissed and reflected the usability problems present in the first prototype which are later mentioned in the focus group.

At the end of this test phase in a controlled environment, all five participants were gathered for the structured focus group composed by seven questions, allowing a better understanding of the issues the user had while using the mobile application, as well as gather suggestions to fix these issues.

Regarding the added value of using the mobile application to stay more informed, the participants stated that adding a mobile component to the +TV4E platform was a good idea, while another participant stated that it could be hard for him to use it in his daily life since he's not used to mobile applications [10].

In regard to the usefulness of being able to access the +TV4E platform outside of their homes, the participants said that they found it useful having the platform available anywhere since they could watch the informative videos as a way to pass the time while also staying informed [10].

When asked if the mobile application should include more information beyond the information provided by the videos, seniores replied that it should also contain information regarding public transports, namely train schedules, information about the weather, local shows, and other events. About "Recommended Videos" tab usefulness, users referred as far as this functionality allows having more control over the videos they can watch, it represents a positive aspect. Seniors also claimed that the videos should be recommended based on their search history. About navigation problems some users said that closing the videos with the backspace was not intuitive and needed to be changed (a possible solution seems to be a small button on the screen to close the video - the final solution considered this hypothesis). The next questions were about the font and icons: the font was considered to be easy to read, however, the users requested that blue colors used in the menu should have more contrast and that the icons must be made more clear (using, for example, a description).

The voice commands were considered very useful and more practical than using the TV remote and all the participants expressed some degree of enthusiasm regarding them.

5.2 Field Trial

The second phase featured four participants and was composed by the field test which lasted eight days, interviews, a SAM and a focus group, in this phase the participants tested the second prototype of the mobile application which included changes proposed by the first sample group.

Platform Usage. Throughout the duration of the field trials, all the videos the participants watched were recorded in a database with the intention of comparing the usage of the platform via the mobile application and the ITV application. The following table (Table 3) presents the viewing method for each video the participants viewed divided into three categories, mobile, TV, and library. Mobile refers to videos watched using the mobile application, which can include watching or re-watching video received on the TV, as well as watching video from the "Recommended Video" tab, TV refers only to videos watched after receiving a notification while watching TV, and Library refer to videos watched or re-watch in the ITV application video library.

As expected, the TV was the primary method for watching informative videos (65%) which is normal since it is the main component of the +TV4E platform while the mobile application serves as a complement to the TV. However, the results reveal that, on average, a considerable number of videos (30%) were watched using the mobile application, which suggests that the users found this new feature of the +TV4E platform useful, which was later confirmed by the interviews and the focus group. It is also interesting that the library was used much less to watch videos (5%) considering it features very similar functionalities to the mobile application. This discrepancy can potentially be

Table 3. Field trial platform' usage.

	ID 1	ID 2	ID 3	ID 4	Total	%
Mobile	12	3	14	10	39	30%
TV	24	4	48	7	83	65%
Library	4	0	3	0	7	5%
Total	40	7	65	17	129	100%

explained because the users found it easier to navigate their videos using the touch interface of the mobile application, or because when watching the TV broadcast they do not want to interrupt it to browse the video library.

Furthermore, it was possible to compare the most popular hours to watch videos on the TV and on the mobile application, which are represented in Fig. 3. Seen videos on TV and Mobile.

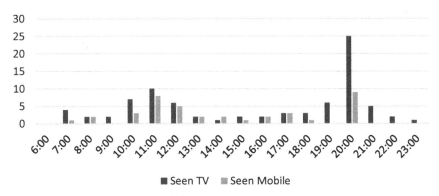

Fig. 3. Seen videos on TV and mobile.

Despite the number of number videos watched on the TV being three times the number of videos watched on the mobile application, the most popular times were very similar for both viewing methods. These results suggest that users mostly used the mobile application in tandem with the ITV application, which means they mostly used the mobile application while they were watching TV, instead of using it as standalone device outside their homes. This goes against the data gathered with the first sample which pointed to the mobile application being most useful when the users are away from their TVs, however it can be since the users did not have enough time to make a habit out of using the +TV4E platform and often remembered to use the mobile application while they were receiving videos on their TVs.

Interviews. In the final day of field testing the users were interviewed regarding their experience with the +TV4E mobile application, these interviews used the same questions as the first sample's focus group for the sake of comparison with the previous results, which inquired the participants regarding their user-experience with the mobile application and asked for suggestions to improve the current prototype. The questions and the user's replies are presented below:

1. Did you consider that the +TV4E mobile application could be an added value for you to stay informed?

- "It is very interesting and could be used on a daily basis, however, it greatly depends on the technological prowess of the senior."
- "It is useful to stay informed since I always have my phone with me."
- "The mobile application should include a greater number and variety of news."
- "It is a good way to stay updated on the news."

2. Do you consider that being able to access the +TV4E platform outside your home is useful?

- "It is useful being able to access the +TV4E platform outside my home."
- "It would be useful for most people."
- "If you have internet access outside your home it is a good way to stay informed."
- "Being able to access the +TV4E platform outside my home is the biggest advantage of the mobile application."

3. Do you think that the mobile application should include more information, such as weather forecasts?

- "It should focus only on news content."
- "It could include information regarding the weather and taxis."
- "Yes, it should include information about cultural events happening near me."
- "It does not need any more content."

4. Do you consider useful having the "Recommended Videos" list?

- "Recommended videos are a useful feature since they provide me with more news."
- "The recommended video list it's very interesting."
- "They are a nice addition since they are not available on the television."
- "It is a very important feature and makes it more interesting."

5. Did you have any problems navigating in the application?

- "Did not have problems navigating the application."
- "Had no problems navigating the application, however, I think the application should come with an instruction manual."
- "Had no problems navigating the application."
- "The mobile application was easy to use."

6. Did you have trouble reading the text in the application or understanding the iconography?

- "Did not have any problems, it was very intuitive to use."
- "Font was easy to read, did not have any problems."
- "Had no problems reading the text or understanding the icons."
- "The icons were easy to understand and the text big enough to read."

7. Did you find the voice commands useful?

- "I found them useful since I was already used to google assistant."
- "Sometimes it was useful, however, it didn't always work properly."
- "I did not use them very much."

The most significant takeaway from the results of these interviews was the absence of complaints regarding the navigation and interface, which were predominant with the previous focus and suggest the changes made to the second prototype addressed most of the issues the users found in the application. Furthermore, it is very positive that this second sample after testing the application for a longer period of time still considered it a useful component of the +TV4E platform and found its portability an important asset. The "Recommended Videos" tab remained a welcomed addition to the platform since it gave the users a bigger sense of control over the platform. The issue that further divided users were the need to include more information in the application, where half of them stated it should only include the informative videos the other half claimed it should include content regarding the weather, taxis and cultural events. This can potentially be addressed by including the required information in a way that does not interfere with the current contents, or by including this information in the form of videos which would blend with the informative videos. Finally, the voice commands were not very popular during the field trials, aside from one user who was already accustomed to using them previously, which suggests this feature needs more work in the future in order to be more appealing to the senior population.

SAM. The SAM scale was applied at the end of the interviews. Figure 4 integrates the mean average score obtained for each item.

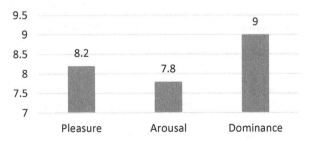

Fig. 4. Second Phase Self-Assessment Manikin results.

The results obtained in this second SAM show a significant improvement in the "Dominance" item, increasing the average by 1.8 points, which can be attributed to the various improvements and fixes made to the first prototype, which aimed to address the biggest complains the users had regarding the navigation in the application. The "Pleasure" item remained roughly the same when compared to the first SAM, dropping from an average of 8.4 to an average of 8.2, while the "Arousal" dropped from an average of 8.6 to an average of 7.8, which can be attributed to the fact that the second sample group tested the application for a much longer period of time and therefore could not maintain the same motivation throughout the duration of the field tests. The results suggest that the overall changes improved the usability of the mobile application.

Focus Group. Finally, the users were gathered for a closing focus regarding their experience with the +TV4E platform, as mentioned previously only the last two questions of the focus group are considered for the purpose of this study, which inquired the participants regarding which aspects they liked or disked about the mobile application and asked for suggestions to improve the current prototype.

The participants found that despite the mobile application being more practical than the iTV application its usage will greatly vary depending on the of senior using the +TV4E platform, implying that only seniors who are already familiar with mobile applications or are willing to learn will make use of it. The biggest advantage of the mobile application was being able to watch informative anywhere at any time. They also stated that the smartphone was their preferred way to look for informative videos they wanted to watch or that caught their attention while watching TV, therefore the mobile application somewhat replaced the role of the video library as a way to catch-up on content they did not watch on the TV. The ability to use the smartphone to watch videos on the TV was praised for the previous reason when the users where at home they rather search for a video on their smartphones and then watch it on the big screen. Aside from the inclusion of more information in application, the only suggestions were the inclusion of push notifications to notify users when a new informative video was available, which the users stated would be a good way to remind them to use the mobile application more often and the addition of an offline mode, so that users could still use the application when they did not have access to the internet.

6   Conclusions

The challenges and opportunities that come up with the ageing process, both at personal and community level, are drawing the attention of several sectors of society. Often, alternatives and solutions are being developed so that ageing is a stage of life marked by high levels of autonomy. This concern is reflected in the efforts undertaken to develop active ageing policies, products and services that promote quality of life in older age. In the last decades, one of the answers to fulfil seniors' needs are the technological innovations that have appeared. Although this type of solutions only make sense if the final user is an active participant in the development solution process, as suggested by the co-creation process. Thus developing software that caters to the needs of the senior population should also be guided by this idea.

Although it is not possible to address the concerns of every senior by keeping the general interface and interaction paradigm simple it is possible to reach a broad audience of older adults. In the case of +TV4E mobile application the results from field trial revealed that many of the issues present in the first prototype were fixed since the results of field trial pointed towards higher levels of usability of the mobile application. Also, it was possible to understand that these levels of usability were achieved mainly due to a design and development process that included target users from the beginning.

Concerning additional features that should be included, some users referred that a notification mechanism to remind the users to watch videos they missed in television or to alert them that new recommendations available in the "Recommended" tab. Additionally, the users stated that it would be a suitable way to remind and motivate people to use the mobile application and not just the iTV application. The voice commands appeared to be a valued feature. The research team plans to introduce them in the ITV application.

Currently, the mobile application was developed to run on Android smartphones, however, to make it more accessible the application also needs to be available for iOS to accommodate iPhone users. Additionally, a version adapted for tablets would also be interesting since several users who participate in this study reported to use a tablet regularly and some even reported to use it more often than their smartphones due to the bigger screen size.

Lastly, an offline mode is also being considered, since currently the application constantly requires an internet connection for all its features and some users pointed this issue as a weak aspect since they report that they are not always connected to the internet. Although this issue was reported as an inconvenience, it is not at all possible to completely make the application work as planned in offline since the +TV4E platform is constantly generating new informative content which needs to be updated at least daily. However, a potential solution to minimize this problem could be having the application download the informative videos to the device when it is connected to the internet, thus allowing users to watch them whether they are connected to the internet or not.

Acknowledgments. The research leading to this work has received funding from Project 3599 – Promover a Produção Científica e Desenvolvimento Tecnológico e a Constituição de Redes Temáticas (3599-PPCDT) and European Commission Funding FEDER (through FCT: Fundação para a Ciência e Tecnologia I.P. under grant agreement no. PTDC/IVC-COM/3206/2014).

References

1. Rosenberg, P., Ross, A., Garçon, L.: WHO Global Forum on Innovations for Ageing Populations. Kobe, Japan (2013)
2. United Nations: World Population Ageing 2015, New York, USA (2015)
3. Teixeira, A., Queirós, A., Rocha, N.P.: Laboratório Vivo de Usabilidade - Living Usability Lab. ARC Publisher (2013)
4. He, W., Goodkind, D., Kowal, P.: An Aging World: 2015 International Population Reports. Washington DC (2016)
5. Kalache, A., Gatti, A.: Active Ageing: a policy framework (2002)
6. Instituto Nacional de Estatística: Projeções de População Residente 2015-2080 (2017)

7. Silva, T., Caravau, H., Campelo, D.: Information needs about public and social services of Portuguese elderly. In: Proceedings of the 3rd International Conference on Information and Communication Technologies for Ageing Well and e-Health, pp. 46–57 (2017)

8. Silva, T., Caravau, H., Ferraz de Abreu, J., Reis, L.: Seniors' info-inclusion through interactive television: results of a field trial. In: Proceedings of the 4th International Conference on Information and Communication Technologies for Ageing Well and e-Health, pp. 134–141 (2018)

9. Silva, T., Campelo, D., Caravau, H., de Abreu, J.F.: Delivering information of general interest through interactive television: a taxonomy of assistance services for the Portuguese elderly. In: Röcker, C., O'Donoghue, J., Ziefle, M., Maciaszek, L., Molloy, W. (eds.) ICT4AWE 2017. CCIS, vol. 869, pp. 191–208. Springer, Cham (2018). https://doi.org/10.1007/978-3-319-93644-4_10

10. Silva, T., Mota, M., Silva, C.: Development and UI/UX testing of an ITV companion application for seniors. In: ICT4AWE 2019 - Proceedings of the 5th International Conference on Information and Communication Technologies for Ageing Well and e-Health, pp. 124–134 (2019)

11. Fredvang, M., Biggs, S.: The Rights of Older Persons: Protection and Gaps Under Human Rights Law (2012)

12. Eisma, R., Dickinson, A., Goodman, J., Syme, A., Tiwari, L., Newell, A.F.: Early user involvement in the development of information technology-related products for older people. Univ. Access Inf. Soc. 3(2), 131–140 (2004)

13. Holzinger, A., Searle, G., Nischelwitzer, A.: On some aspects of improving mobile applications for the elderly. In: Stephanidis, C. (ed.) UAHCI 2007. LNCS, vol. 4554, pp. 923–932. Springer, Heidelberg (2007). https://doi.org/10.1007/978-3-540-73279-2_103

14. Hawthorn, D.: Designing Effective Interfaces for Older Users. The University of Waikato, Hamilton (2006)

15. Pereira, L.: Princípios orientadores de design de interfaces para aplicações ITV orientadas para seniores portugueses. Universidade do Porto (2013)

16. Reis, L., Caravau, H., Silva, T., Almeida, P.: Automatic CREATion of TV content to integrate in seniors viewing activities. In: Abásolo, M.J., Almeida, P., Pina Amargós, J. (eds.) jAUTI 2016. CCIS, vol. 689, pp. 32–46. Springer, Cham (2017). https://doi.org/10.1007/978-3-319-63321-3_3

17. Verona, S.M., Da Cunha, C., Pimenta, G.C., Buriti, M.D.A.: Percepção do idoso em relação à Internet. Temas em Psicol., vol. 14, pp. 189–197, October 2006

18. Silva, T., Mota, M., Hernández, C., De Abreu, J.F.: Automatic creation of informative TV videos to be delivered through iTV: a system architecture. Procedia Comput. Sci. 121, 584–591 (2017)

19. Campelo, D., Silva, T., Abreu, J.: Recommending personalized informative contents on iTV. In: Adjunct Publication of the 2017 ACM International Conference on Interactive Experiences for TV and Online Video - TVX 2017, Adjunct, pp. 99–103 (2017)

20. Nielsen, J., Molich, R.: Heuristic evaluation of user interfaces. In: Proceedings of the SIGCHI Conference on Human Factors in Computing Systems Empowering People - CHI 1990, pp. 249–256 (1990)

Author Index

Printed in the United States
By Bookmasters